Breast Cancer, Fertility Preservation and Reproduction

Nicoletta Biglia • Fedro Alessandro Peccatori
Editors

Breast Cancer, Fertility Preservation and Reproduction

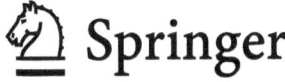
Springer

Editors

Nicoletta Biglia
Department of Obstetrics and Gynaecology
University of Torino School of Medicine
Mauriziano Umberto I Hospital
Torino
Italy

Fedro Alessandro Peccatori
Fertility and Procreation Unit
Istituto Europeo di Oncologia
Milano
Italy

ISBN 978-3-319-17277-4   ISBN 978-3-319-17278-1   (eBook)
DOI 10.1007/978-3-319-17278-1

Library of Congress Control Number: 2015939681

Springer Cham Heidelberg New York Dordrecht London

Printed on acid-free paper

Springer International Publishing AG Switzerland is part of Springer Science+Business Media (www.springer.com)

Foreword

The incidence of breast cancer in young and premenopausal women is increasing in Europe and in the USA. At the same time, a trend towards delaying pregnancy to later in life has been observed and many women will receive a diagnosis of breast cancer before completing their families.

Although a diagnosis of cancer is distressing at any age, in young women it is fraught with several unique challenges including its impact on reproduction.

Women with a history of breast neoplasm should be given the possibility to conceive and get mother, particularly if they have not completed their planned family.

Thanks to advances in early diagnosis and treatment, the cure rate at present is very high and many young women will ask to their gynaecologists and oncologists a great many questions about the feasibility and safety of attempting a pregnancy after breast cancer. Will pregnancy eventually impair my prognosis? When can I start trying and get pregnant? Is it mandatory to carry on the endocrine treatment up to the scheduled end? What is the impact of chemotherapy? Are there any risks for the newborn? Do I have a higher risk of abortion because of my disease? Will I be able to breastfeed? And many more.

Nicoletta Biglia and Fedro Peccatori with this book provide us invaluable "state-of-the-art" answers to the above questions, but this is only the tip of the iceberg.

They raise and discuss many more points.

Fertility preservation is among the most prominent ones, because it requires a prompt decision and shifts the time for dealing with the problem from the end of the treatment to a short time window before starting chemotherapy.

The advent of assisted reproduction techniques within the oncology field has made fertility preservation a viable option, but several studies have shown that fertility counselling remains inadequate and lacks of a standardised approach.

In clinical practice, gynaecologists and oncologists are frequently faced with women who need to be thoroughly informed about the available fertility preservation techniques but, possibly because of a kind of discomfort and lack of knowledge, eventually leave fertility concerns poorly addressed.

This book will provide them with the most updated scientific knowledge on this subject and hopefully will motivate them to be proactive in addressing the fertility preservation issue.

Finally, the authors bring to our attention and discuss in depth a new and fascinating challenge, for those of us dealing everyday with young women with breast cancer: the debated issue of fertility preservation and preimplantation genetic diagnosis in BRCA mutation carriers.

I am proud of having stimulated the authors to edit this book!

Turin, Italy   Piero Sismondi

Contents

Epidemiology of Breast Cancer in Young Women

Fabio Parazzini, Antonella Villa, Giampiero Polverino,
Stefania Noli, and Giovanna Scarfone

Breast cancer is the most frequent cancer among women and it is the second leading cause of cancer death around the world. It is the most commonly diagnosed cancer in women between the ages of 25 and 39 (CANCERMondial http://ci5.iarc.fr/CI5plus/ci5plus.htm).

Breast cancer cases observed in young women have some clinical epidemiological and genetic characteristics that differ from those observed among older ones.

Breast cancer in young women has an aggressive course of clinical presentation [1], a higher rate of germline mutation in BRCA 1&2 [2], distinct estrogen and progesterone receptor expression, and over-expression of human epidermal growth factor receptor 2 (HER2) [3, 4]. Further, they are different also in the epidemiological profile.

In this chapter, we reviewed the epidemiology of breast cancer among women aged 40 years or less.

1.1 Frequency

In the USA, the SEER report estimates the risk of developing breast cancer in 10-year age intervals. According to the current report, the risk that a woman will be diagnosed with breast cancer during the next 10 years, starting at the age of 30 is 1 in about 230 (www.cancer.gov/cancertopics).

The incidence rate of breast cancer among women aged 20–24 years in the USA is 1.5 cases per 100,000 women and about 50 per 100,000 women among women

F. Parazzini (✉) • A. Villa • G. Polverino • S. Noli • G. Scarfone
Dipartimento di Scienze Cliniche e di Comunità, Dipartimento Materno Infantile, IRCCS Policlinico, Università di Milano, Via Commenda 12, 20122 Milan, Italy
e-mail: fabio.parazzini@unimi.it; giovanna.scarfone@unimi.it; antonella.villa@unimi.it; giampiero.polverino@unimi.it

© Springer International Publishing Switzerland 2015
N. Biglia, F.A. Peccatori (eds.), *Breast Cancer, Fertility Preservation and Reproduction*, DOI 10.1007/978-3-319-17278-1_1

aged 35 years (Breast Cancer Facts & Figures 2011–2012). In Italy, the rate is about 35/100,000 women aged 35 years [5].

Considering the US population, about 7 % of all cases are diagnosed before age 40, 2.4 % are diagnosed before age 35, and 1 % diagnosed before age 30 [6].

Of all cancers diagnosed among women, more than 40 % is breast cancer by the age of 40, 20 % by the age of 30, and slightly more than 2 % by 20 years of age.

1.1.1   Geographical Differences

The incidence of breast cancer in young women is lower in developed countries [7] in comparison with developing ones.

However, the incidence of breast cancer among young women in the low-risk population of the South Asian countries is higher [8].

1.1.2   Temporal Trends

Data on the temporal trends of breast cancer incidence in young women are scant and limited [9].

Some recent studies have suggested that the incidence of breast cancer in young [4, 10, 11] and premenopausal women [12, 13] increased in Europe and the USA.

A study from different countries of Europe showed an overall increase of 1.19 % per year from 1990 to 2008 [11]. The incidence increased more consistently among women under 35 compared to the 36–40 years cohort.

A study from France reported an increase during the period of 1983–2002 [10].

Similar findings also emerged from analysis conducted in Asian countries. An analysis including data from tumor registries in China, Japan, Singapore, and the Philippines considering the calendar period 1970–2002 showed that the trend in incidence for the age group 16–29 increased from 0.45 to 1.07 corresponding to an AAPC of 2.8 % (95%CI 1.9, 3.7). In age group 30–40, the incidence ranged from 13.3 in year 1970 to 24.8 in year 2002 corresponding to an AAPC of 2.7 % (95 % CI 2.3, 3.1). There were two statistically significant changing points in the regression line for the age groups 30–40 and 16–40: one point in the year 1975 with an APC of 6.1 (5.1, 7.1) and the other in 1985 with an APC of 0.4 % (0.01) [13].

Considering developing countries, a study conducted in Brazil reported an annual increase of 5.22 % in the incidence of breast cancer among age group 30–40 years during the period 1988–2003 [14].

Different trends have been observed in the same country in different ethnic groups.

For example in the USA, white women who were 40 years or older had a higher rate of breast cancer than black women in the same age group, but among younger women black women had higher rates. Otherwise, the annual percentage change in invasive breast cancer incidence increased only among white women younger than 40 years.

Other racial and ethnic groups had lower incidence rates than non-Hispanic white women for all three age groups and did not exhibit the crossover pattern observed among black women, although IRRs were slightly higher among younger than older Hispanic, API, and AI/AN women.

Any change in trend of any disease, especially breast cancer, can be attributed to either a true increase due to an underlying change of some risk factors, the result of an improvement in the quality of data collection or screening practice.

Along this line, part of these different trends could be explained by different frequency among countries and ethnic group of screening procedures. A younger age at onset among the Asian population has been reported and it has been attributed to a cohort effect that has been decreasing in recent decades [15].

1.1.3 Breast Cancer in Pregnancy

Among young women, a specific topic is the incidence of the disease during pregnancy or in women who have recently delivered.

Breast cancer is generally reported to be the most common pregnancy-related cancer in all the populations. It accounts for about one-third of all pregnancy-related cancers. Its incidence mirrors the incidence of breast cancer among nonpregnant women of the same age class. In developed countries, the risk of breast cancer diagnosis in pregnancy or during the first year after delivery is about 1:3,000 pregnancies.

1.2 Clinical and Histopathological Characteristics of Breast Cancer Among Young Women

It is generally suggested that breast cancer tends to be more aggressive in young women. This finding could be due to different factors such as delayed diagnosis and consequent advanced disease stage and/or unfavorable tumor characteristics [16].

1.2.1 Stage

It is commonly reported that young breast cancer patients are diagnosed with more advanced stages.

In fact, breast cancer cases in young women have larger tumors, more frequent nodal involvement, and are more likely to be diagnosed with stage II or III cancer than older patients [17].

This may be at least in part due to the fact that younger women are not screened for breast cancer. In fact, mammography is not recommended in women less than 40 years.

Further, young women are often less likely to seek early medical advice, leading to later detection often at more advanced stages [18].

Pregnancy is another reason to delay diagnosis, since pregnant women may tend underreport breast nodules.

1.2.2 Histotypes

The tumors diagnosed in young women have different characteristics than those in older ones. Young women have a lower rate of ductal carcinoma in situ. This may be due to a detection bias, since, as previously underlined, women under 40 years of age do not have screening mammograms.

1.2.3 Grading

Further, tumors in young women are more likely to be high grade and to have high proliferation index.

Among young women, lymphovascular invasion is more common than among older ones [19].

1.2.4 Hormone Receptor/HER2 Expression

Many studies have shown that young women with breast cancer have more commonly hormone receptor (HR) negative tumors. Otherwise, HER2 is overexpressed [3].

Further, young women are likely to be diagnosed with HR+/HER2- subtype of breast cancer, followed by triple negative, HR+/HER2+, and HR-/HER2+ subtypes. Multiple studies demonstrated the overrepresentation of triple-negative breast cancers in young patients particularly in African Americans [1].

In a retrospective study of 700 breast tumors conducted by Anders et al. women younger than 45 years were less likely to have estrogen receptor-positive disease, and more likely to have grade 3 tumors, nodal metastasis, and larger primary breast tumors [20].

1.3 Genetics

The role of hereditary is of great relevance among young women [21].

In women <35 years of age with breast cancer, the frequency of a BRCA1 or BRCA2 gene mutation is about 10 %, which is more than ten times the frequency in the general population [2].

BRCA1 and BRCA2 gene mutations are observed in about 65–75 % of all inherited breast cancer cases. The presence of these mutations markedly increases (about tenfold) the relative risk of breast cancer. BRCA1-associated breast cancer is more likely to involve higher-grade tumors, basal-like subtypes, and triple-negative breast cancer [2].

Patients between the ages of 30 and 34 with ER-negative, high-grade tumors have a 26–28 % chance of having a deleterious BRCA1 mutation [22].

p53 mutation (including the Li–Fraumeni syndrome), PTEN mutation (Cowden's disease), and Lynch syndromes have been also strictly associated with the risk of breast cancer in young women [23, 24].

Anders et al. [20] identified 367 gene sets that could differentiate tumors in young women from tumors in older women (young, ≤45 years; and older, ≥65 years).

1.4   Risk Factors

Most of the risk factors for breast cancer in young women are similar to those for tumors observed in older patients [25].

However, specific studies addressing risk factors for breast cancer in young women have suggested that the effect of oral contraceptive use and pregnancy is more related to cases observed in young women [26]. Conversely, body mass index is more strongly related to the risk in older women.

In this section, we briefly review the evidence on risk factors for breast cancer that have a different role among young and older women.

1.4.1   Race and Ethnicity

The incidence of breast cancer is the highest in the non-Hispanic white population. When stratified by age, incidence rates are similar for non-Hispanic whites and African Americans between the ages of 30 and 49 years. However, in patients younger than 40 years specifically, African American females have the highest relative incidence of breast cancer [27, 28].

In women over 45, breast cancer is more common in whites than blacks. However, black women under age 35 have more than twice the incidence of invasive breast cancer and three times the breast cancer mortality of young white women [6].

In contrast, Native American women aged 20–44 have a lower incidence of breast cancer (relative risk [RR]=0.7) compared to the general population.

1.4.2   Family History

A positive family history of breast cancer is the main risk factor among young women. Women under 35 years of age with a positive family history of the diseases have 3–4 times higher risk of the disease than women without family history [29].

1.4.3   Contralateral Breast Cancer

Young women with breast cancer have an about doubled increased risk of contralateral breast cancer [30]. The estimated cumulative risk is about 13 % in a 10-year period [31].

Continuing exposure to risk factors, radiation for the treatment of the initial breast cancer, and genetic profile can at least in part explain the increased risk of contralateral breast cancer in these patients [32].

1.4.4 Hormonal Factors

Inconsistent results were published regarding age at menarche and breast cancer risk [33]. Some studies reported that younger age at menarche increased breast cancer risk only in premenopausal women, while some reported increased risk only for postmenopausal women [33, 34, 35]. In some previous studies, age at menarche was found to be associated with both pre-and postmenopausal breast cancer, while in another studies, it had no association with either pre- or postmenopausal breast cancer [33, 34, 35]. In this study, early onset of menarche was found to be associated with both pre- and postmenopausal patients as the majority of patients in either groups attained puberty at an age of <12 years. The median age of menarche worldwide is 14 years (range 11 to 18 years). Some studies done on Indian women showed that the risk of both premenopausal and postmenopausal breast cancer decreased with delay in the onset of menarche [36].

Hormonal risk factors are somewhat different for women aged less than 35 years in comparison to older women.

Pregnancy plays a protective role on the risk of breast cancer on long term. However, it increases the risk immediately after delivery. Thus delayed childbirth (first child after age 30 years) is a risk factor for breast cancer in older women, but early childbearing seems to be a risk factor for developing breast cancer before the age of 35 years.

A similar effect has been suggested for oral contraceptives (OC): current use of OC increases the risk, but previous use decreases the risk. Along this line, recent oral contraceptive use is a risk factor for early-onset breast cancer, particularly for estrogen receptor (ER)-negative tumors.

1.4.5 Body Mass Index

There is evidence that breast cancer risk is positively associated with body mass index in postmenopausal women. A large population-based study evaluating approximately 50,000 women indicated that the combination of obesity, high-energy (caloric) intake, and sedentary lifestyle is a risk factor in premenopausal women [37].

1.4.6 Physical Activity

Participation in recreational or occupational physical activity may decrease estrogen levels, reducing body fat, and, with extreme exercise, reducing the frequency of ovulation. Further physical activity may increase levels of sex hormone binding globulin (SHBG), which would reduce bioavailable estrogens [38]. Increased physical activity also reduces insulin resistance and hyperinsulinemia, which has been hypothesized to be related to breast cancer [38].

Along this line, intense physical activity has been associated with a decreased breast cancer risk in premenopausal women [39].

1.4.7   Diet and Selected Micronutrient Intake

Among dietary factors, a high intake of certain fruits and vegetables (e.g., tomatoes) has been associated with a decreased risk of breast cancer in young women [40].

No relationship has been found between calcium/vitamin D intake and the risk of postmenopausal breast cancer, but several studies suggest that high vitamin D intake, with or without calcium, may protect against premenopausal breast cancer [41–43].

It has been suggested that among premenopausal women, 400 IU vitamin D and 1,000 mg calcium daily lower mean breast density and breast density is associated with the risk of breast cancer in premenopausal women [44].

1.4.8   Miscellaneous

Other risk factors for breast cancer in premenopausal women include a history of prior mantle irradiation for Hodgkin lymphoma [29].

Conclusion

Although a diagnosis of cancer is distressing at any age, the diagnosis of a breast cancer in young women is fraught with several unique challenges due to its impact of self-imaging, the relation with the partner, reproduction, and in general the life expectance.

Since breast cancer in young women is not a rare condition, special focus should be given to the identification of women at high (familiar/genetic) risk for this condition. Due to the observation that breast cancer in young women is more frequently diagnosed at higher stage, early diagnosis, in the perspective of the clinical epidemiology, remains a priority.

References

1. Tichy JR, Lim E, Anders CK. Breast cancer in adolescents and young adults: a review with a focus on biology. J Natl Compr Canc Netw. 2013;11:1060–9.
2. Malone KE, Daling JR, Neal C, Suter NM, O'Brien C, Cushing-Haugen K, Jonasdottir TJ, Thompson JD, Ostrander EA. Frequency of BRCA1/BRCA2 mutations in a population-based sample of young breast carcinoma cases. Cancer. 2000;88:1393–402.
3. Bleyer A, Barr R, Hayes-Lattin B, Thomas D, Ellis C, Anderson B. The distinctive biology of cancer in adolescents and young adults. Nat Rev Cancer. 2008;8:288–98.
4. Gabriel CA, Domchek SM. Breast cancer in young women. Breast Cancer Res. 2010;12:212.
5. AIRT Working Group. Italian cancer figures–report 2006: 1. Incidence, mortality and estimates. Epidemiol Prev. 30;2006:8–10, 12–28, 30–101 passim.
6. Anders CK, Fan C, Parker JS, Carey LA, Blackwell KL, Klauber-DeMore N, Perou CM. Breast carcinomas arising at a young age: unique biology or a surrogate for aggressive intrinsic subtypes? J Clin Oncol. 2011;29:e18–20.
7. Brinton LA, Sherman ME, Carreon JD, Anderson WF. Recent trends in breast cancer among younger women in the United States. J Natl Cancer Inst. 2008;100:1643–8.

8. Pradhananga KK, Baral M, Shrestha BM. Multi-institution hospital-based cancer incidence data for Nepal: an initial report. Asian Pac J Cancer Prev. 2009;10:259–62.
9. Afsharfard A, Mozaffar M, Orang E, Tahmasbpour E. Trends in epidemiology, clinical and histopathological characteristics of breast cancer in Iran: results of a 17 year study. Asian Pac J Cancer Prev. 2013;14:6905–11.
10. Colonna M, Delafosse P, Uhry Z, Poncet F, Arveux P, Molinie F, Cherie-Challine L, Grosclaude P. Is breast cancer incidence increasing among young women? An analysis of the trend in France for the period 1983–2002. Breast. 2008;17:289–92.
11. Leclere B, Molinie F, Tretarre B, Stracci F, Daubisse-Marliac L, Colonna M. Trends in incidence of breast cancer among women under 40 in seven European countries: a GRELL cooperative study. Cancer Epidemiol. 2013;37:544–9.
12. Cardoso F, Loibl S, Pagani O, Graziottin A, Panizza P, Martincich L, Gentilini O, Peccatori F, Fourquet A, Delaloge S, Marotti L, Penault-Llorca F, Kotti-Kitromilidou AM, Rodger A, Harbeck N. The European Society of Breast Cancer Specialists recommendations for the management of young women with breast cancer. Eur J Cancer. 2012;48:3355–77.
13. Keramatinia A, Mousavi-Jarrahi SH, Hiteh M, Mosavi-Jarrahi A. Trends in incidence of breast cancer among women under 40 in Asia. Asian Pac J Cancer Prev. 2014;15:1387–90.
14. Freitas Jr R, Freitas NM, Curado MP, Martins E, Silva CM, Rahal RM, Queiroz GS. Incidence trend for breast cancer among young women in Goiania, Brazil. Sao Paulo Med J. 2010;128:81–4.
15. Mousavi-Jarrrahi SH, Kasaeian A, Mansori K, Ranjbaran M, Khodadost M, Mosavi-Jarrahi A. Addressing the younger age at onset in breast cancer patients in Asia: an age-period-cohort analysis of fifty years of quality data from the international agency for research on cancer. ISRN Oncol. 2013;2013:429862.
16. Bharat A, Aft RL, Gao F, Margenthaler JA. Patient and tumor characteristics associated with increased mortality in young women (< or =40 years) with breast cancer. J Surg Oncol. 2009;100:248–51.
17. Gajdos C, Tartter PI, Bleiweiss IJ, Bodian C, Brower ST. Stage 0 to stage III breast cancer in young women. J Am Coll Surg. 2000;190:523–9.
18. Friedman LC, Kalidas M, Elledge R, Dulay MF, Romero C, Chang J, Liscum KR. Medical and psychosocial predictors of delay in seeking medical consultation for breast symptoms in women in a public sector setting. J Behav Med. 2006;29:327–34.
19. Thapa B, Singh Y, Sayami P, Shrestha UK, Sapkota R, Sayami G. Breast cancer in young women from a low risk population in Nepal. Asian Pac J Cancer Prev. 2013;14:5095–9.
20. Anders CK, Hsu DS, Broadwater G, Acharya CR, Foekens JA, Zhang Y, Wang Y, Marcom PK, Marks JR, Febbo PG, Nevins JR, Potti A, Blackwell KL. Young age at diagnosis correlates with worse prognosis and defines a subset of breast cancers with shared patterns of gene expression. J Clin Oncol. 2008;26:3324–30.
21. Reyna C, Lee MC. Breast cancer in young women: special considerations in multidisciplinary care. J Multidiscip Healthc. 2014;7:419–29.
22. Lakhani SR, Van De Vijver MJ, Jacquemier J, Anderson TJ, Osin PP, McGuffog L, Easton DF. The pathology of familial breast cancer: predictive value of immunohistochemical markers estrogen receptor, progesterone receptor, HER-2, and p53 in patients with mutations in BRCA1 and BRCA2. J Clin Oncol. 2002;20:2310–8.
23. Kleihues P, Schauble B, Hausen A, Esteve J, Ohgaki H. Tumors associated with p53 germline mutations: a synopsis of 91 families. Am J Pathol. 1997;150:1–13.
24. He X, Arrotta N, Radhakrishnan D, Wang Y, Romigh T, Eng C. Cowden syndrome-related mutations in PTEN associate with enhanced proteasome activity. Cancer Res. 2013;73:3029–40.
25. Anders CK, Johnson R, Litton J, Phillips M, Bleyer A. Breast cancer before age 40 years. Semin Oncol. 2009;36:237–49.
26. Daling JR, Malone KE, Voigt LF, White E, Weiss NS. Risk of breast cancer among young women: relationship to induced abortion. J Natl Cancer Inst. 1994;86:1584–92.

27. DeSantis C, Howlader N, Cronin KA, Jemal A. Breast cancer incidence rates in U.S. women are no longer declining. Cancer Epidemiol Biomarkers Prev. 2011;20:733–9.
28. DeSantis C, Ma J, Bryan L, Jemal A. Breast cancer statistics, 2013. CA Cancer J Clin. 2014;64:52–62.
29. Althuis MD, Brogan DD, Coates RJ, Daling JR, Gammon MD, Malone KE, Schoenberg JB, Brinton LA. Breast cancers among very young premenopausal women (United States). Cancer Causes Control. 2003;14:151–60.
30. Hartman M, Czene K, Reilly M, Bergh J, Lagiou P, Trichopoulos D, Adami HO, Hall P. Genetic implications of bilateral breast cancer: a population based cohort study. Lancet Oncol. 2005;6:377–82.
31. Lee KD, Chen SC, Chan CH, Lu CH, Chen CC, Lin JT, Chen MF, Huang SH, Yeh CM, Chen MC. Increased risk for second primary malignancies in women with breast cancer diagnosed at young age: a population-based study in Taiwan. Cancer Epidemiol Biomarkers Prev. 2008;17:2647–55.
32. Kollias J, Ellis IO, Elston CW, Blamey RW. Clinical and histological predictors of contralateral breast cancer. Eur J Surg Oncol. 1999;25:584–9.
33. Kwan ML, Kushi LH, Weltzien E, Maring B, Kutner SE, Fulton RS, Lee MM, Ambrosone CB, Caan BJ. Epidemiology of breast cancer subtypes in two prospective cohort studies of breast cancer survivors. Breast Cancer Res. 2009;11:R31.
34. Pathy NB, Yip CH, Taib NA, Hartman M, Saxena N, Iau P, Bulgiba AM, Lee SC, Lim SE, Wong JE, Verkooijen HM. Breast cancer in a multi-ethnic Asian setting: results from the Singapore-Malaysia hospital-based breast cancer registry. Breast. 2011;20 Suppl 2:S75–80.
35. Butt Z, Haider SF, Arif S, Khan MR, Ashfaq U, Shahbaz U, Bukhari MH. Breast cancer risk factors: a comparison between pre-menopausal and post-menopausal women. J Pak Med Assoc. 2012;62:120–4.
36. Sandhu DS, Sandhu S, Karwasra RK, Marwah S. Profile of breast cancer patients at a tertiary care hospital in north India. Indian J Cancer. 2010;47:16–22.
37. Silvera SA, Jain M, Howe GR, Miller AB, Rohan TE. Energy balance and breast cancer risk: a prospective cohort study. Breast Cancer Res Treat. 2006;97:97–106.
38. Macfarlane GJ, Lowenfels AB. Physical activity and colon cancer. Eur J Cancer Prev. 1994;3:393–8.
39. Slattery ML, Edwards S, Murtaugh MA, Sweeney C, Herrick J, Byers T, Giuliano AR, Baumgartner KB. Physical activity and breast cancer risk among women in the southwestern United States. Ann Epidemiol. 2007;17:342–53.
40. Do MH, Lee SS, Kim JY, Jung PJ, Lee MH. Fruits, vegetables, soy foods and breast cancer in pre- and postmenopausal Korean women: a case–control study. Int J Vitam Nutr Res. 2007;77:130–41.
41. Abbas S, Linseisen J, Chang-Claude J. Dietary vitamin D and calcium intake and premenopausal breast cancer risk in a German case–control study. Nutr Cancer. 2007;59:54–61.
42. Braverman AS. Evidence that high calcium and vitamin D intake decrease the risk of breast cancer in premenopausal women: implications for breast cancer prevention and screening. South Med J. 2007;100:1061–2.
43. Lin J, Manson JE, Lee IM, Cook NR, Buring JE, Zhang SM. Intakes of calcium and vitamin D and breast cancer risk in women. Arch Intern Med. 2007;167:1050–9.
44. Berube S, Diorio C, Masse B, Hebert-Croteau N, Byrne C, Cote G, Pollak M, Yaffe M, Brisson J. Vitamin D and calcium intakes from food or supplements and mammographic breast density. Cancer Epidemiol Biomarkers Prev. 2005;14:1653–9.

Managing Breast Cancer in Young Women

Joyce G. Habib and Hatem A. Azim Jr.

2.1   Introduction

Breast cancer arising in young women is relatively uncommon constituting around 5–7 % of women diagnosed in the Western World [1, 2]. The prevalence is higher in the developing world, with up to 20 % of patients diagnosed below the age of 40 in Africa and the Middle East [3, 4].

Breast cancer in young women differs in several aspects from tumors diagnosed in older patients. Women ≤40 tend to have advanced disease at diagnosis, typically presenting with large palpable, often multifocal tumors and exhibiting higher prevalence of lymphatic involvement and nodal spread [1, 5, 6]. Moreover, young age at breast cancer diagnosis has consistently been shown to be an independent predictor of worse outcome in both early and late stage disease [1, 6–10]. This likely provides an explanation for the trends observed in clinical practice favoring mastectomy and adjuvant chemotherapy use in this patient population despite lack of proven recurrence or survival benefit justifying a more aggressive treatment approach [11–18].

It is unclear whether the adverse clinical and histologic features of breast cancer in young patients can entirely account for their increased risk of relapse and disease-related mortality. Despite lack of differences in stage-adjusted short-term survival in younger compared to older women [19], studies with long-term follow-up have revealed that survival disparities are more prominent in early rather than late stage disease [1, 20], emphasizing the precedence of tumor biology over clinical stage as predictor of outcome in this disease [21].

Higher rates of hormone-receptor negative and HER2-overexpressing tumors occur in younger patients [1, 3]. Other adverse histologic features seen in this patient population include high tumor grade, poor differentiation, and

J.G. Habib • H.A. Azim Jr. (✉)
Department of Medicine, BrEAST Data Centre,
Boulevard de Waterloo, 121, 1000 Brussels, Belgium
e-mail: Joyce.habib@bordet.be; Hatem.azim@bordet.be

© Springer International Publishing Switzerland 2015
N. Biglia, F.A. Peccatori (eds.), *Breast Cancer, Fertility Preservation and Reproduction*, DOI 10.1007/978-3-319-17278-1_2

lymphovascular invasion [1, 5, 22–26]. Using gene expression profiling, young patients were shown to have higher incidence of basal-like tumors compared to their older counterparts [27, 28]. In addition, unlike their older counterparts, luminal-B subtype constitutes the majority of the ER-positive population in young patients [29]. Nevertheless, recent evidence further points to the existence of subtype-independent differential expression of several biological processes related to apoptosis, PI3k signaling, stem cells, stroma-related genes, and others underlying the unique biology of breast cancer in this specific patient population [28].

In this chapter, we will be discussing in detail different aspects related to the management of breast cancer arising in young women. Acknowledging their unique biology, and guarded prognosis, it is reasonable to think that their management strategies should be somehow tailored. In addition, young women often have different perspectives of quality of life and survivorship issues compared to their older counterparts, which should be taken into account when discussing treatment expectations.

2.2 Diagnostic Work-Up: Specific Considerations in Young Patients

2.2.1 Diagnostic Imaging

When compared to older patients, young patients tend to present more frequently with locally advanced disease including larger tumor size ($\geq$T3) and higher rates of nodal involvement [1]. This is likely due to a combination of multiple factors including lack of routine screening, decreased sensitivity of mammography, and low index of suspicion in symptomatic younger patients.

The work-up of young patients without or unknown genetic predisposition does not differ from that in older patients. Mammography and ultrasonography remain the diagnostic studies of choice with ultrasound being the preferred first-line imaging modality in pregnant woman or those aged <30 years old presenting with symptoms or suspicious clinical examination [30]. As in older patients, palpable breast masses or suspicious axillary adenopathy in young patients should also prompt a referral for biopsy even in the absence of radiographic disease.

The sensitivity of digital mammography is superior to that of film mammography in dense breasts; therefore, its use for diagnostic purposes may be preferable in young patients [31, 32]. The improved diagnostic accuracy of novel mammographic techniques such as tomosynthesis over digital mammography particularly in dense breasts may be promising for young patients; however, at this time there is little data to support their use.

MRI is more sensitive than mammography in tumor size assessment and detection of multifocal disease and is relatively unaffected by breast density [33]. However, MRI is not routinely used in the diagnostic setting in young women without genetic predisposition given the lack of convincing evidence for improvement in local recurrence, distant recurrence, or reoperation rates [34–37]. The utility of

MRI imaging for detecting synchronous contralateral breast cancer also remains an area of controversy regardless of the patient's age. In high-risk women with known BRCA deleterious mutations or increased risk of breast malignancy based on family history, MRI is recommended and routinely used despite uncertainty regarding survival advantage in this setting [38].

2.2.2 Genetic Counseling

Regardless of the underlying breast cancer subtype, genetic counseling referral should be an integral part of the evaluation of all newly diagnosed young patients. Testing for hereditary breast/ovarian cancer predisposition is recommended for all women diagnosed at age ≤45 due to higher prevalence of deleterious BRCA mutations even among unselected patients [39, 40]. Genetic referral and testing should ideally occur early on during the initial disease work-up as it bears implications for both the decision and timing of prophylactic contralateral mastectomy and/or prophylactic bilateral salpingo-oophorectomy, if needed [41]. Women with breast cancer before the age of 30 and no detectable BRCA mutation have an estimated 4–8 % likelihood of harboring a TP53 germline mutation which is further increased with personal or family history of Li–Fraumeni syndrome-related cancer [42–44]. These considerations provide the basis for expert consensus guidelines endorsing TP53 testing either concurrently or after negative BRCA testing in women with breast cancer diagnosed at age ≤35 [40].

2.3 Surgical Management and Radiotherapy-Related Considerations in Young Patients

2.3.1 Surgery

Pooled data from randomized controlled trials and patient-based cohorts demonstrate a two- to fourfold increase in locoregional recurrence risk with breast conservation surgery in women ≤40 when compared to older patients [45–49]. However, patients included in some of the earlier studies were treated prior to the routine use of radiation boost or the advent of modern chemotherapy and adjuvant trastuzumab. Improvements in surgical techniques, radiotherapy, systemic therapy, and the use of adjuvant HER2-targeted therapy have contributed to decreasing local recurrence rates in this patient population. For instance, the 5-year locoregional recurrence rates (LRR) in subgroups of patients ≤40 old at diagnosis treated in the Netherlands during the periods 1988–1998, 1999–2005, and 2006–2010 were found to be 9.8 %, 5.9 %, and 3.3 %, respectively [50]. In a recent series, no differences in LRR were observed in breast cancer patients ≤40 years old at diagnosis treated with either breast conservation surgery or mastectomy [12]. These changing statistics are at odds with the current trends observed in clinical practice. The increasing rates of ipsilateral and contralateral prophylactic mastectomies among young women with breast cancer are likely driven by patients' perception of an associated survival benefit [11, 18, 51, 52]. However, current data suggest that long-term survival is not adversely affected in women who opt for breast conservation surgery as opposed to mastectomy [13, 15, 53]. Similarly, contralateral prophylactic mastectomy, in the absence of BRCA mutation, has not been associated with improvement in OS in younger patients and should not be routinely recommended. Discussion regarding risks and benefits related to this procedure should be held between both patient and provider before a decision is made [54, 55].

In young patients seeking breast conservation surgery, there is no evidence to support that more widely clear margin than no ink on tumor affects LRR [56]. There is likewise no evidence to suggest a higher false-negative rate for sentinel lymph node biopsy (SLNB) performed in young patients; therefore, indications for SLNB and surgical management of patients with sentinel node involvement are the same across all age groups [57]. In women meeting ACOSOG Z0011 inclusion criteria (T1-2 disease, clinically negative axilla and up to two positive sentinel lymph nodes), breast conservation surgery with tangential whole-breast radiotherapy appears to be sufficient and hence axillary lymph node dissection and radiation can be omitted without adverse impact on outcome [58, 59].

2.3.2 Radiotherapy

Women with early stage breast cancer undergoing breast conservation surgery should receive conventional tangential whole-breast irradiation (45–50.4 Gy at fractionated doses of 1.8–2.0 Gy delivered 5 days per week) with 10–16 Gy boost delivered to the tumor bed. The local recurrence relative risk reduction achieved with the addition of boost is similar regardless of age; however, for younger women at higher baseline risk for local relapse, the benefit in terms of absolute risk reduction is expected to be higher [60, 61]. Only 20–30 % of women included in trials comparing hypofractionated to conventional radiation (RT) therapy were <50 years old. Apart from age, other characteristics of patients included in these studies (primarily T1–T2 tumors, node-negative, low-grade disease) suggest a lower baseline recurrence risk compared to the one typically seen in young breast cancer patients with high-grade or locally advanced disease. The effect of age on locoregional recurrence was reported in one of these trials showing no difference in local control in women younger than 50 compared to those ≥50 [62]. However, since no further age stratification was performed, it is unclear whether similar results can be expected in women <40 as opposed to women 40–49 years old. High-grade disease, despite being underrepresented in hypofractionated RT trials, was shown to be associated with higher local relapse when treated with hypofractionated RT (10-year risk of IBTR 15.6 % vs 4.7 % for hypofractionated vs. conventional RT, respectively) [62]. Thus, in keeping with ASTRO guidelines, the use of hypofractionated RT in young patients with breast cancer is currently not recommended but may be considered in selected patients in the absence of high-grade disease and if meeting criteria of patients enrolled in these trials [63]. Accelerated partial breast irradiation (APBI) is not indicated in young patients outside a clinical trial given that published data and current guidelines only apply to women older than 50–60 [63, 64]. Results of ongoing phase III studies such NSABP B-39/RTOG 0413, RAPID (randomized trial of accelerated partial breast irradiation), GEC-ESTRO should provide answers on the potential use of these modalities in younger patients [65].

Young age at breast cancer diagnosis has been associated with an increased risk of local relapse after mastectomy and involvement of the internal mammary chain [66]. Thus, post-mastectomy radiotherapy with inclusion of the internal mammary chain may be considered and decision should be made on an individual basis after discussion of risks and benefits with the patient.

2.4   Adjuvant Systemic Therapy

2.4.1   Chemotherapy and Trastuzumab

As discussed earlier, young age at breast cancer diagnosis has been considered as a surrogate for high-risk disease and is often used as an inclusion criterion in adjuvant chemotherapy trials. Based on this, clinicians traditionally have lower threshold for administering adjuvant chemotherapy in younger patients, including those with ER-positive, HER2-negative disease. However, it should be noted that results of the latest EBCTG meta-analysis have indicated that the use of anthracycline and taxane-based adjuvant chemotherapy was associated with similar proportional risk reduction in breast cancer recurrence and mortality irrespective of age [67]. This suggests that age alone should not be used to guide the use of chemotherapy.

Genomic signatures have emerged as useful tools to improve prognostications but also may guide the need for adjuvant chemotherapy in patients with ER-positive disease. Existing evidence suggest that these genomic assays provide similar prognostic information irrespective of age [28]. Evidence on the utility of these signatures as predictive markers for chemotherapy benefit is limited to Oncotype DX, based on retrospective evaluation of two prospective studies [68, 69]. In a cohort from National Surgical Adjuvant Breast and Bowel Project (NSABP) B-14, no significant benefit was seen with the addition of chemotherapy to hormonal therapy in patients with lymph node-negative breast cancer premenopausal patients with low recurrence risk scores [68]. The same finding was observed in NSABP-B20 in postmenopausal patients with node-positive disease [69]. The ongoing prospective randomized clinical trial, TAILORx, will confirm the clinical utility of this assay, in particularly evaluating the benefit of chemotherapy in patients with intermediate risk. In addition, this trial will provide valuable information on the value of Oncotype DX in younger patients as well. Although the 70-gene signature panel, Mammaprint, has been validated as prognostic tool, its clinical utility on whether it could guide therapeutic decisions remains unproven with the ongoing study, Microarray in Node-Negative Disease May Avoid Chemotherapy (MINDACT), intended to clarify this question [70–73].

There is no evidence to suggest that young women with TNBC or HER2-positive disease derive more benefit from adjuvant chemotherapy compared to older patients [14, 74, 75]. When pooled adjuvant chemotherapy trial data were analyzed looking only at ER-poor disease and excluding adjuvant tamoxifen use, both absolute and relative risk reduction in breast cancer recurrence and mortality were comparable in women <50 vs. those ≥50 years old [74]. While these results should be interpreted with caution, in view of different measurement techniques and definition of ER positivity in the individual included studies, similar findings were also reported in an analysis of a more recent patient cohort [14].

In HER2-positive disease, a retrospective analysis of the adjuvant study HERA has shown that young age (≤40 years old) was not associated with higher risk of early relapse. In addition, young patients appear to derive similar benefit from adjuvant trastuzumab compared to their older counterparts [75]. In practice, administration of adjuvant chemotherapy in young patients presenting with breast cancer subtypes, associated with high relapse risk such as HER2-positive breast cancer or TNBC, does not pose challenge to clinicians. Instead, the dilemma arise when these patients present with T1a/b, N0 triple-negative, or HER2-overexpressing breast cancer, a population relatively underrepresented in adjuvant clinical trials. In these situations, clinicians often face the difficult task of determining at which age or tumor size cut-off withholding adjuvant chemotherapy would not adversely impact the patient's long-term prognosis. Higher recurrence risk and cancer-specific mortality in women <35–50 years old has been reported in several studies in T1a-b N0 HER2-positive and TNBC regardless of whether they received adjuvant chemotherapy or not [16, 17, 76–78]. Nevertheless, it remains unclear to this date whether higher rates of adjuvant chemotherapy use in young patients with small node-negative, triple-negative, or HER2-overexpressing tumors would actually translate into a meaningful reduction in recurrence risk or mortality in this patient population [16, 17].

2.4.2 Endocrine Therapy

Five years of tamoxifen has been long considered the standard adjuvant endocrine therapy for young breast cancer patients. The EBCTG updated analysis shows that 5 years of adjuvant tamoxifen reduces the relative risk of recurrence and death at 15 years by approximately 40 % and 30 %, respectively, independent of age [79]. However, recent data have suggested that extended treatment beyond 5 years could be a superior approach. In the MA17 trial, the addition of 5 years of letrozole after completion of 5 years of tamoxifen was shown to significantly reduce recurrence rates mainly in women who were premenopausal at the time of tamoxifen therapy initiation [80]. In addition, results from the two largest extended adjuvant tamoxifen studies (ATLAS and aTTom) have demonstrated lower recurrence risk and survival advantage for 10 years over 5 years of adjuvant tamoxifen [81, 82].

Several guidelines have incorporated these findings and recommend 10 years of adjuvant tamoxifen as a valid treatment option for women who are still premenopausal after completion of 5 years of tamoxifen or newly diagnosed patients who are likely to remain premenopausal after 5 years of adjuvant tamoxifen. It should be noted though that only ATLAS included women <45 years old with less than 50 % of them being premenopausal (9–10 % with ER-positive disease in each treatment arm). Assuming that the proportional risk reduction in mortality from extended adjuvant therapy is the same across all age groups, it remains modest at best with uncertainty that it will carry over when this practice is implemented in the community. Compliance is dependent on duration of therapy and compliance rates in ATLAS and aTTOM were noted to decrease from 80 % at 7–8 years to 60 % at 10 years. In the community setting where significantly lower adherence rates are observed particularly among younger patients, further extension of duration of adjuvant hormonal therapy may not replicate the same benefits seen in these studies [83, 84].

One important question that needs to be addressed is whether there are subsets of young breast cancer patients that could potentially derive more benefit from extended adjuvant hormonal therapy. In recent years, several gene expression signatures have shown to be good predictors of late recurrence in hormone-receptor positive breast cancer such as Breast Cancer Index (BCI), Endopredict, and PAM50 (ROR) [85–87]. Therefore, one important area of investigation would be to determine the extent of benefit from extended adjuvant endocrine therapy in patients classified as high risk for late relapse by these assays.

Another unanswered question concerns the role of ovarian ablation in the adjuvant setting in young breast cancer patients. Young women developing chemotherapy-induced amenorrhea for ≥ 6 months have been shown to have improved survival, underscoring the validity of inducing amenorrhea at least for a period of time [88]. Nevertheless, the benefit from ovarian ablation in premenopausal women in the adjuvant setting remains uncertain and to date we lack generalized consensus on whether ovarian ablation should be routinely used [89]. Ovarian ablation after anthracycline and non-anthracycline-based adjuvant chemotherapy similarly has not resulted in improved outcome overall, despite an observed trend for benefit in terms of recurrence and DFS in premenopausal women <40 with ER-positive disease [90–92]. This was also seen in a meta-analysis of individual patient data enrolled in these studies [93]. However keeping in mind that the majority of these studies have not compared ovarian ablation to or after chemotherapy with tamoxifen included in both arms, it is unclear whether the benefit from ovarian ablation is superior to tamoxifen alone.

Lately several studies have attempted to address this question by combining ovarian ablation to either tamoxifen or aromatase inhibitors in the adjuvant setting in hormone-receptor positive breast cancer [94–97] (Table 2.1).

At present time, there is no role for aromatase inhibitors with or without ovarian ablation in patients who remain premenopausal after 5 years of tamoxifen. For patients who become menopausal during/after completion of adjuvant tamoxifen, a switching or extended adjuvant strategy may be considered. Ovarian ablation in combination with aromatase inhibitor may be considered as upfront adjuvant therapy in premenopausal patients in view of SOFT/TEXT combined analysis however,

Table 2.1 Summary of phase III randomized trials evaluating the role of ovarian ablation with tamoxifen and/or aromatase inhibitors

Trial	Patient population characteristics	Study design	Median follow-up	DFS (HR, 95 % CI)	OS (HR, 95 % CI)
ABCSG-12 [94, 96]	1,803 premenopausal women. No adjuvant chemotherapy Median age 45 Stage I/II (75 % T1 tumors, 67 % N0).	Randomized, open-label, two-by-two factorial design Goserelin + tamoxifen vs. goserelin + anastrazole +/− zoledronic acid for 3 years	62 months	HR 1.08, 95 % CI 0.81–1.44; p=0.591	HR 1.75, 95 % CI 1.08–2.83; p=0.02)
SOFT (IBCSG 24–02) [95, 98]	3,066 premenopausal women. 53.5 % received chemotherapy Median age 40 chemotherapy arm, 46 no chemotherapy arm) Stage I–III (59 % T1 tumors, 66 % N0)	Randomized, open-label 1:1:1 ratio Tamoxifen vs. triptorelin + tamoxifen vs. triptorelin + exemestane for 5 years	68 months	Combined analysis Tamoxifen + triptorelin vs. exemestane + triptorelin: HR 0.72, 95 % CI 0.60–0.86; p<0.001) Tamoxifen + triptorelin vs. tamoxifen alone: HR 0.83, 95 % CI 0.66–1.04; p=0.10	HR 1.14, 95 % CI 0.86–1.51; p=0.37). Data not mature
TEXT (IBCSG 25–02) [95]	2,672 premenopausal patients 39.6 % received adjuvant chemotherapy Median age 45 chemotherapy arm, 43 no chemotherapy arm) Stage I–III (66 % T1 tumors, 52 % N0)	Randomized, open-label 1:1 ratio Triptorelin + tamoxifen vs. triptorelin + exemestane for 5 years	68 months		
E-3193, INT-0142 [97]	345 premenopausal women. No adjuvant chemotherapy Median age 45 Stage I–II (91% T1 tumors, 100 % N0)	Randomized, open-label 1:1 ratio Tamoxifen vs. tamoxifen + ovarian ablation For 5 years Ovarian ablation included LHRH agonist (36 %), surgical (42 %), or RT (13 %) ovarian ablation	9.9 years	HR 1.17, 95 % CI 0.64–2.12; p=0.62) No difference in OS between study arms. HR 1.19, 95 % CI 0.52–2.70; p=0.67)	HR 1.19, 95 % CI 0.52–2.70; p=0.67

longer follow-up is needed at this point. Only INT0142 had long-term follow-up; however, the study is underpowered for survival analysis due to early closure as a result of poor accrual. Nevertheless, the sample size was achieved for patient-related outcomes with results indicating, as expected more menopausal symptoms and decline in sexual activity in the ovarian ablation arm [97]. Another concern is the worse outcome of the ovarian ablation + anastrazole arm compared to ovarian ablation + tamoxifen arm of the ABCSG-12 trial. Several hypotheses have been proposed to explain these results including short treatment duration (3 years) and also lack of HER2 status assessment. More recently, an unplanned analysis of the ABCSG-12 trial suggested that the poor outcome of the anastrazole arm is only restricted to overweight population, which constituted around 30 % of the study population [99]. These results raise questions regarding the use of aromatase inhibitors in overweight/obese premenopausal women. This becomes more complicated when compliance issues are also considered. Higher rates of musculoskeletal and gynecologic side effects with aromatase inhibitors may further compromise low compliance rates in this patient population. Conversely, potential incomplete ovarian suppression due to non-adherence with scheduled LHRH administration coupled with continued use of aromatase inhibitor therapy in a patient population considered at higher risk for recurrence also warrants careful consideration. Given these issues and taking into account the relative short follow-up in SOFT/TEXT, awaiting mature data from these two trials seems more cautious at this time.

2.4.3   Neoadjuvant Therapy

Data comparing the impact of neoadjuvant chemotherapy in younger compared to older patients are scarce. Evidence suggests that younger patients with TNBC seem to derive the more benefit from neoadjuvant chemotherapy with higher rates of pathologic complete response (pCR) reported in women <35 compared to older patients [100, 101]. However, a pooled neoadjuvant trial analysis did not find a difference in DFS according to age when patients achieved pCR to neoadjuvant chemotherapy. As such, age per se should not guide the use of neoadjuvant chemotherapy.

Similarly, limited data regarding the use of neoadjuvant hormonal therapy are available. Non-randomized studies and more recently a randomized double-blind Study of Tamoxifen or Arimidex, combined with Goserelin acetate, to compare Efficacy and safety (STAGE) trial have looked at ovarian ablation combined with an aromatase inhibitor in the neoadjuvant setting [102–104]. In STAGE, neoadjuvant goserelin combined with either tamoxifen or anastrazole for 24 weeks prior to definitive surgery was compared in premenopausal patients with T2N0M0 ER-positive breast cancer with the primary endpoint being best overall response (complete and partial response) assessed clinically [102]. Significantly higher clinical response rates (complete and partial) were seen with the aromatase inhibitor-LHRH combination (70 % vs. 50 %); however, no differences in pCR rates were noted between study arms. Interpretation of these findings and the applicability of neoadjuvant endocrine therapy in young patients in the absence of long-term outcome data are limited at this time.

2.4.4 Metastatic Breast Cancer

The choice of chemotherapy and HER2-targeted therapy is guided by the same principles irrespective of age [105]. There is also no evidence to suggest that combination cytotoxic chemotherapy in young patients with metastatic breast cancer offers survival or quality of life benefit over sequential monotherapy [106].

Options for endocrine therapy in metastatic breast cancer in premenopausal patients include single-agent tamoxifen and, unlike in the adjuvant setting, the combination of tamoxifen with an LHRH analog shown to offer survival advantage in this setting [107]. The combination of LHRH agonist with aromatase inhibitor has been evaluated in small studies either as first- or second-line therapy in the metastatic setting [108–114]. Very limited data are available on the use of fulvestrant and everolimus in premenopausal patients [115]. Therefore, they should not be currently considered: although there is no reason to think that they would not be as effective as in postmenopausal patients and is worthy of investigation in young patients.

2.5 Take-Home Messages

Management of young patients with breast cancer still poses challenge to clinicians with several questions unanswered at this time. Reconciling the divergent findings of neoadjuvant, adjuvant, and non-randomized studies in small node-negative HER2-positive or TNBC is needed to better understand the prognostic significance of younger age in these breast cancer subtypes. In ER-positive disease, better stratification of late relapse risk in young patients could help optimize the use of extended adjuvant hormonal therapy in this patient population. The role of ovarian ablation in the adjuvant setting in combination with tamoxifen or an aromatase inhibitor with or without prior adjuvant chemotherapy needs to be better defined and mature data from SOFT/TEXT should provide further insight into this matter. Exploiting the biology of ER-positive breast cancer in young patients to tailor adjuvant chemotherapy is also the subject of ongoing research. Evaluation of drugs such as everolimus with potential activity against deregulated molecular signaling associated with breast cancer in young patients may potentially lead to decreased indiscriminate cytotoxic chemotherapy use in this patient population. Correlating underlying tumor biology, treatment, and outcome in these studies will be important to design meaningful targeted therapy. The contribution of stromal signaling to carcinogenesis and tumor progression in young patients is increasingly being recognized and future research will also help determine the significance of stromal signaling and its influence of recurrence and outcome in younger patients.

References

1. Gnerlich JL, Deshpande AD, Jeffe DB, Sweet A, White N, Margenthaler JA. Elevated breast cancer mortality in women younger than age 40 years compared with older women is attributed to poorer survival in early-stage disease. J Am Coll Surg. 2009;208(3):341–7.
2. DeSantis C, Ma J, Bryan L, Jemal A. Breast cancer statistics, 2013. CA Cancer J Clin. 2014;64(1):52–62.
3. Akarolo-Anthony SN, Ogundiran TO, Adebamowo CA. Emerging breast cancer epidemic: evidence from Africa. Breast Cancer Res BCR. 2010;12 Suppl 4:S8.
4. El Saghir NS, Khalil MK, Eid T, El Kinge AR, Charafeddine M, Geara F, et al. Trends in epidemiology and management of breast cancer in developing Arab countries: a literature and registry analysis. Int J Surg Lond Engl. 2007;5(4):225–33.
5. Copson E, Eccles B, Maishman T, Gerty S, Stanton L, Cutress RI, et al. Prospective observational study of breast cancer treatment outcomes for UK women aged 18–40 years at diagnosis: the POSH study. J Natl Cancer Inst. 2013;105(13):978–88.
6. Fredholm H, Eaker S, Frisell J, Holmberg L, Fredriksson I, Lindman H. Breast cancer in young women: poor survival despite intensive treatment. PLoS One. 2009;4(11):e7695.
7. Albain KS, Allred DC, Clark GM. Breast cancer outcome and predictors of outcome: are there age differentials? J Natl Cancer Inst Monogr. 1994;16:35–42.
8. Han W, Kang SY. Korean Breast Cancer Society. Relationship between age at diagnosis and outcome of premenopausal breast cancer: age less than 35 years is a reasonable cut-off for defining young age-onset breast cancer. Breast Cancer Res Treat. 2010;119(1):193–200.
9. Swanson GM, Lin CS. Survival patterns among younger women with breast cancer: the effects of age, race, stage, and treatment. J Natl Cancer Inst Monogr. 1994;16:69–77.
10. Chung M, Chang HR, Bland KI, Wanebo HJ. Younger women with breast carcinoma have a poorer prognosis than older women. Cancer. 1996;77(1):97–103.
11. Rosenberg S. Choosing mastectomy over lumpectomy: factors associated with surgical decisions in young women with breast cancer. J Clin Oncol 31. 2013(Suppl; Abstr 6507).
12. Buckley J. Recurrence rates and long-term survival in women diagnosed with breast cancer at age 40 and younger. J Clin Oncol 29. 2011(Suppl 27; Abstr 70).
13. Cao JQ, Truong PT, Olivotto IA, Olson R, Coulombe G, Keyes M, et al. Should women younger than 40 years of age with invasive breast cancer have a mastectomy?: 15-year outcomes in a population-based cohort. Int J Radiat Oncol Biol Phys. 2014;90(3):509–17.
14. Sheridan W, Scott T, Caroline S, Yvonne Z, Vanessa B, David V, et al. Breast cancer in young women: have the prognostic implications of breast cancer subtypes changed over time? Breast Cancer Res Treat. 2014;147(3):617–29.
15. Mahmood U, Morris C, Neuner G, Koshy M, Kesmodel S, Buras R, et al. Similar survival with breast conservation therapy or mastectomy in the management of young women with early-stage breast cancer. Int J Radiat Oncol Biol Phys. 2012;83(5):1387–93.
16. Migdady Y, Sakr BJ, Sikov WM, Olszewski AJ. Adjuvant chemotherapy in T1a/bN0 HER2-positive or triple-negative breast cancers: application and outcomes. Breast Edinb Scotl. 2013;22(5):793–8.
17. Olszewski AJ, Migdady Y, Boolbol SK, Klein P, Boachie-Adjei K, Sakr BJ, et al. Effects of adjuvant chemotherapy in HER2-positive or triple-negative pT1ab breast cancers: a multi-institutional retrospective study. Breast Cancer Res Treat. 2013;138(1):215–23.
18. Mahmood U, Hanlon AL, Koshy M, Buras R, Chumsri S, Tkaczuk KH, et al. Increasing national mastectomy rates for the treatment of early stage breast cancer. Ann Surg Oncol. 2013;20(5):1436–43.
19. Keegan THM, Press DJ, Tao L, DeRouen MC, Kurian AW, Clarke CA, et al. Impact of breast cancer subtypes on 3-year survival among adolescent and young adult women. Breast Cancer Res BCR. 2013;15(5):R95.
20. Xiong Q, Valero V, Kau V, Kau SW, Taylor S, Smith TL, et al. Female patients with breast carcinoma age 30 years and younger have a poor prognosis: the M.D. Anderson Cancer Center experience. Cancer. 2001;92(10):2523–8.

21. Azim HA Jr, Partridge AH. Biology of breast cancer in young women. Breast Cancer Res. 2014;16:427.
22. Gajdos C, Tartter PI, Bleiweiss IJ, Bodian C, Brower ST. Stage 0 to stage III breast cancer in young women. J Am Coll Surg. 2000;190(5):523–9.
23. Winchester DP, Osteen RT, Menck HR. The National Cancer Data Base report on breast carcinoma characteristics and outcome in relation to age. Cancer. 1996;78(8):1838–43.
24. Gonzalez-Angulo AM, Broglio K, Kau S-W, Eralp Y, Erlichman J, Valero V, et al. Women age<or=35 years with primary breast carcinoma: disease features at presentation. Cancer. 2005;103(12):2466–72.
25. Keegan THM, DeRouen MC, Press DJ, Kurian AW, Clarke CA. Occurrence of breast cancer subtypes in adolescent and young adult women. Breast Cancer Res BCR. 2012;14(2):R55.
26. Collins LC, Marotti JD, Gelber S, Cole K, Ruddy K, Kereakoglow S, et al. Pathologic features and molecular phenotype by patient age in a large cohort of young women with breast cancer. Breast Cancer Res Treat. 2012;131(3):1061–6.
27. Anders CK, Hsu DS, Broadwater G, Acharya CR, Foekens JA, Zhang Y, et al. Young age at diagnosis correlates with worse prognosis and defines a subset of breast cancers with shared patterns of gene expression. J Clin Oncol Off J Am Soc Clin Oncol. 2008;26(20):3324–30.
28. Azim HA Jr, Michiels S, Bedard PL, Singhal SK, Criscitiello C, Ignatiadis M, et al. Elucidating prognosis and biology of breast cancer arising in young women using gene expression profiling. Clin Cancer Res Off J Am Assoc Cancer Res. 2012;18(5):1341–51.
29. Azim HA Jr, Azim H. Breast cancer arising at a young age: do we need to define a cut-off? Breast Edinb Scotl. 2013;22(6):1007–8.
30. Loving VA, DeMartini WB, Eby PR, Gutierrez RL, Peacock S, Lehman CD. Targeted ultrasound in women younger than 30 years with focal breast signs or symptoms: outcomes analyses and management implications. AJR Am J Roentgenol. 2010;195(6):1472–7.
31. Pisano ED, Gatsonis C, Hendrick E, Yaffe M, Baum JK, Acharyya S, et al. Diagnostic performance of digital versus film mammography for breast-cancer screening. N Engl J Med. 2005;353(17):1773–83.
32. Pisano ED, Hendrick RE, Yaffe MJ, Baum JK, Acharyya S, Cormack JB, et al. Diagnostic accuracy of digital versus film mammography: exploratory analysis of selected population subgroups in DMIST. Radiology. 2008;246(2):376–83.
33. Sardanelli F, Giuseppetti GM, Panizza P, Bazzocchi M, Fausto A, Simonetti G, et al. Sensitivity of MRI versus mammography for detecting foci of multifocal, multicentric breast cancer in Fatty and dense breasts using the whole-breast pathologic examination as a gold standard. AJR Am J Roentgenol. 2004;183(4):1149–57.
34. Peters NHGM, van Esser S, van den Bosch MA, Storm RK, Plaisier PW, van Dalen T, et al. Preoperative MRI and surgical management in patients with nonpalpable breast cancer: the MONET – randomised controlled trial. Eur J Cancer Oxf Engl 1990. 2011;47(6):879–86.
35. Turnbull L, Brown S, Harvey I, Olivier C, Drew P, Napp V, et al. Comparative effectiveness of MRI in breast cancer (COMICE) trial: a randomised controlled trial. Lancet. 2010;375(9714):563–71.
36. Houssami N, Turner R, Morrow M. Preoperative magnetic resonance imaging in breast cancer: meta-analysis of surgical outcomes. Ann Surg. 2013;257(2):249–55.
37. McGhan LJ, Wasif N, Gray RJ, Giurescu ME, Pizzitola VJ, Lorans R, et al. Use of preoperative magnetic resonance imaging for invasive lobular cancer: good, better, but maybe not the best? Ann Surg Oncol. 2010;17 Suppl 3:255–62.
38. Morrow M, Waters J, Morris E. MRI for breast cancer screening, diagnosis, and treatment. Lancet. 2011;378(9805):1804–11.
39. Golshan M, Miron A, Nixon AJ, Garber JE, Cash EP, Iglehart JD, et al. The prevalence of germline BRCA1 and BRCA2 mutations in young women with breast cancer undergoing breast-conservation therapy. Am J Surg. 2006;192(1):58–62.
40. National Comprehensive Cancer Network. Breast Cancer (Version 3.2014). http://www.nccn.org/professionals/physician_gls/pdf/breast.pdf. Accessed 10 Nov 2014.
41. Wevers MR, Aaronson NK, Verhoef S, Bleiker EMA, Hahn DEE, Kuenen MA, et al. Impact of rapid genetic counselling and testing on the decision to undergo immediate or delayed

prophylactic mastectomy in newly diagnosed breast cancer patients: findings from a randomised controlled trial. Br J Cancer. 2014;110(4):1081–7.

42. Gonzalez KD, Noltner KA, Buzin CH, Gu D, Wen-Fong CY, Nguyen VQ, et al. Beyond Li Fraumeni Syndrome: clinical characteristics of families with p53 germline mutations. J Clin Oncol Off J Am Soc Clin Oncol. 2009;27(8):1250–6.

43. McCuaig JM, Armel SR, Novokmet A, Ginsburg OM, Demsky R, Narod SA, et al. Routine TP53 testing for breast cancer under age 30: ready for prime time? Fam Cancer. 2012;11(4): 607–13.

44. Mouchawar J, Korch C, Byers T, Pitts TM, Li E, McCredie MRE, et al. Population-based estimate of the contribution of TP53 mutations to subgroups of early-onset breast cancer: Australian Breast Cancer Family Study. Cancer Res. 2010;70(12):4795–800.

45. Botteri E, Bagnardi V, Rotmensz N, Gentilini O, Disalvatore D, Bazolli B, et al. Analysis of local and regional recurrences in breast cancer after conservative surgery. Ann Oncol Off J Eur Soc Med Oncol ESMO. 2010;21(4):723–8.

46. Voogd AC, Nielsen M, Peterse JL, Blichert-Toft M, Bartelink H, Overgaard M, et al. Differences in risk factors for local and distant recurrence after breast-conserving therapy or mastectomy for stage I and II breast cancer: pooled results of two large European randomized trials. J Clin Oncol Off J Am Soc Clin Oncol. 2001;19(6):1688–97.

47. De Bock GH, van der Hage JA, Putter H, Bonnema J, Bartelink H, van de Velde CJ. Isolated loco-regional recurrence of breast cancer is more common in young patients and following breast conserving therapy: long-term results of European Organisation for Research and Treatment of Cancer studies. Eur J Cancer Oxf Engl 1990. 2006;42(3):351–6.

48. Fisher ER, Anderson S, Tan-Chiu E, Fisher B, Eaton L, Wolmark N. Fifteen-year prognostic discriminants for invasive breast carcinoma: National Surgical Adjuvant Breast and Bowel Project Protocol-06. Cancer. 2001;91(8 Suppl):1679–87.

49. Early Breast Cancer Trialists' Collaborative Group (EBCTCG), Darby S, McGale P, Correa C, Taylor C, Arriagada R, et al. Effect of radiotherapy after breast-conserving surgery on 10-year recurrence and 15-year breast cancer death: meta-analysis of individual patient data for 10,801 women in 17 randomised trials. Lancet. 2011;378(9804):1707–16.

50. Van Laar C, van der Sangen MJC, Poortmans PMP, Nieuwenhuijzen GA, Roukema JA, Roumen RMH, et al. Local recurrence following breast-conserving treatment in women aged 40 years or younger: trends in risk and the impact on prognosis in a population-based cohort of 1143 patients. Eur J Cancer Oxf Engl 1990. 2013;49(15):3093–101.

51. Pesce CE, Liederbach E, Czechura T, Winchester DJ, Yao K. Changing surgical trends in young patients with early stage breast cancer, 2003 to 2010: a report from the National Cancer Data Base. J Am Coll Surg. 2014;219(1):19–28.

52. McGuire KP, Santillan AA, Kaur P, Meade T, Parbhoo J, Mathias M, et al. Are mastectomies on the rise? A 13-year trend analysis of the selection of mastectomy versus breast conservation therapy in 5865 patients. Ann Surg Oncol. 2009;16(10):2682–90.

53. Bantema-Joppe EJ, de Munck L, Visser O, Willemse PHB, Langendijk JA, Siesling S, et al. Early-stage young breast cancer patients: impact of local treatment on survival. Int J Radiat Oncol Biol Phys. 2011;81(4):e553–9.

54. Pesce C, Liederbach E, Wang C, Lapin B, Winchester DJ, Yao K. Contralateral prophylactic mastectomy provides no survival benefit in young women with estrogen receptor-negative breast cancer. Ann Surg Oncol. 2014;21(10):3231–9.

55. Portschy PR, Kuntz KM, Tuttle TM. Survival outcomes after contralateral prophylactic mastectomy: a decision analysis. J Natl Cancer Inst. 2014;106(8):dju160.

56. Moran MS, Schnitt SJ, Giuliano AE, Harris JR, Khan SA, Horton J, et al. Society of Surgical Oncology-American Society for Radiation Oncology consensus guideline on margins for breast-conserving surgery with whole-breast irradiation in stages I and II invasive breast cancer. J Clin Oncol Off J Am Soc Clin Oncol. 2014;32(14):1507–15.

57. Lyman GH, Giuliano AE, Somerfield MR, Benson AB, Bodurka DC, Burstein HJ, et al. American Society of Clinical Oncology guideline recommendations for sentinel lymph node biopsy in early-stage breast cancer. J Clin Oncol Off J Am Soc Clin Oncol. 2005; 23(30):7703–20.

58. Giuliano AE, Hunt KK, Ballman KV, Beitsch PD, Whitworth PW, Blumencranz PW, et al. Axillary dissection vs no axillary dissection in women with invasive breast cancer and sentinel node metastasis: a randomized clinical trial. JAMA. 2011;305(6):569–75.
59. Giuliano AE, McCall L, Beitsch P, Whitworth PW, Blumencranz P, Leitch AM, et al. Locoregional recurrence after sentinel lymph node dissection with or without axillary dissection in patients with sentinel lymph node metastases: the American College of Surgeons Oncology Group Z0011 randomized trial. Ann Surg. 2010;252(3):426–32; discussion 432–3.
60. Jones HA, Antonini N, Hart AAM, Peterse JL, Horiot J-C, Collin F, et al. Impact of pathological characteristics on local relapse after breast-conserving therapy: a subgroup analysis of the EORTC boost versus no boost trial. J Clin Oncol Off J Am Soc Clin Oncol. 2009;27(30):4939–47.
61. Bartelink H, Horiot J-C, Poortmans PM, Struikmans H, Van den Bogaert W, Fourquet A, et al. Impact of a higher radiation dose on local control and survival in breast-conserving therapy of early breast cancer: 10-year results of the randomized boost versus no boost EORTC 22881–10882 trial. J Clin Oncol Off J Am Soc Clin Oncol. 2007;25(22):3259–65.
62. Whelan TJ, Pignol J-P, Levine MN, Julian JA, MacKenzie R, Parpia S, et al. Long-term results of hypofractionated radiation therapy for breast cancer. N Engl J Med. 2010;362(6):513–20.
63. Smith BD, Bentzen SM, Correa CR, Hahn CA, Hardenbergh PH, Ibbott GS, et al. Fractionation for whole breast irradiation: an American Society for Radiation Oncology (ASTRO) evidence-based guideline. Int J Radiat Oncol Biol Phys. 2011;81(1):59–68.
64. Polgár C, Van Limbergen E, Pötter R, Kovács G, Polo A, Lyczek J, et al. Patient selection for accelerated partial-breast irradiation (APBI) after breast-conserving surgery: recommendations of the Groupe Européen de Curiethérapie-European Society for Therapeutic Radiology and Oncology (GEC-ESTRO) breast cancer working group based on clinical evidence (2009). Radiother Oncol J Eur Soc Ther Radiol Oncol. 2010;94(3):264–73.
65. Njeh CF, Saunders MW, Langton CM. Accelerated Partial Breast Irradiation (APBI): a review of available techniques. Radiat Oncol Lond Engl. 2010;5:90.
66. Veronesi U, Cascinelli N, Bufalino R, Morabito A, Greco M, Galluzzo D, et al. Risk of internal mammary lymph node metastases and its relevance on prognosis of breast cancer patients. Ann Surg. 1983;198(6):681–4.
67. Early Breast Cancer Trialists' Collaborative Group (EBCTCG), Peto R, Davies C, Godwin J, Gray R, Pan HC, et al. Comparisons between different polychemotherapy regimens for early breast cancer: meta-analyses of long-term outcome among 100,000 women in 123 randomised trials. Lancet. 2012;379(9814):432–44.
68. Paik S, Shak S, Tang G, Kim C, Baker J, Cronin M, et al. A multigene assay to predict recurrence of tamoxifen-treated, node-negative breast cancer. N Engl J Med. 2004;351(27):2817–26.
69. Albain KS, Barlow WE, Shak S, Hortobagyi GN, Livingston RB, Yeh I-T, et al. Prognostic and predictive value of the 21-gene recurrence score assay in postmenopausal women with node-positive, oestrogen-receptor-positive breast cancer on chemotherapy: a retrospective analysis of a randomised trial. Lancet Oncol. 2010;11(1):55–65.
70. Van de Vijver MJ, He YD, van't Veer LJ, Dai H, Hart AAM, Voskuil DW, et al. A gene-expression signature as a predictor of survival in breast cancer. N Engl J Med. 2002;347(25):1999–2009.
71. Buyse M, Loi S, van't Veer L, Viale G, Delorenzi M, Glas AM, et al. Validation and clinical utility of a 70-gene prognostic signature for women with node-negative breast cancer. J Natl Cancer Inst. 2006;98(17):1183–92.
72. Mook S, Schmidt MK, Weigelt B, Kreike B, Eekhout I, van de Vijver MJ, et al. The 70-gene prognosis signature predicts early metastasis in breast cancer patients between 55 and 70 years of age. Ann Oncol Off J Eur Soc Med Oncol ESMO. 2010;21(4):717–22.
73. Cardoso F, Van't Veer L, Rutgers E, Loi S, Mook S, Piccart-Gebhart MJ. Clinical application of the 70-gene profile: the MINDACT trial. J Clin Oncol Off J Am Soc Clin Oncol. 2008;26(5):729–35.

74. Early Breast Cancer Trialists' Collaborative Group (EBCTCG), Clarke M, Coates AS, Darby SC, Davies C, Gelber RD, et al. Adjuvant chemotherapy in oestrogen-receptor-poor breast cancer: patient-level meta-analysis of randomised trials. Lancet. 2008;371(9606):29–40.
75. Partridge AH, Gelber S, Piccart-Gebhart MJ, Focant F, Scullion M, Holmes E, et al. Effect of age on breast cancer outcomes in women with human epidermal growth factor receptor 2-positive breast cancer: results from a herceptin adjuvant trial. J Clin Oncol Off J Am Soc Clin Oncol. 2013;31(21):2692–8.
76. Tai P, Cserni G, Van De Steene J, Vlastos G, Voordeckers M, Royce M, et al. Modeling the effect of age in T1-2 breast cancer using the SEER database. BMC Cancer. 2005;5:130.
77. Gonzalez-Angulo AM, Litton JK, Broglio KR, Meric-Bernstam F, Rakkhit R, Cardoso F, et al. High risk of recurrence for patients with breast cancer who have human epidermal growth factor receptor 2-positive, node-negative tumors 1 cm or smaller. J Clin Oncol Off J Am Soc Clin Oncol. 2009;27(34):5700–6.
78. Hanrahan EO, Gonzalez-Angulo AM, Giordano SH, Rouzier R, Broglio KR, Hortobagyi GN, et al. Overall survival and cause-specific mortality of patients with stage T1a, bN0M0 breast carcinoma. J Clin Oncol Off J Am Soc Clin Oncol. 2007;25(31):4952–60.
79. Early Breast Cancer Trialists' Collaborative Group (EBCTCG), Davies C, Godwin J, Gray R, Clarke M, Cutter D, et al. Relevance of breast cancer hormone receptors and other factors to the efficacy of adjuvant tamoxifen: patient-level meta-analysis of randomised trials. Lancet. 2011;378(9793):771–84.
80. Goss PE, Ingle JN, Martino S, Robert NJ, Muss HB, Livingston RB, et al. Impact of pre-menopausal status at breast cancer diagnosis in women entered on the placebo-controlled NCIC CTG MA17 trial of extended adjuvant letrozole. Ann Oncol Off J Eur Soc Med Oncol ESMO. 2013;24(2):355–61.
81. Davies C, Pan H, Godwin J, Gray R, Arriagada R, Raina V, et al. Long-term effects of continuing adjuvant tamoxifen to 10 years versus stopping at 5 years after diagnosis of oestrogen receptor-positive breast cancer: ATLAS, a randomised trial. Lancet. 2013;381(9869): 805–16.
82. Gray R. aTTom: long-term effects of continuing adjuvant tamoxifen to 10 years versus stopping at 5 years in 6,953 women with early breast cancer. J Clin Oncol 31. 2013(Suppl; Abstr 5).
83. Murphy CC, Bartholomew LK, Carpentier MY, Bluethmann SM, Vernon SW. Adherence to adjuvant hormonal therapy among breast cancer survivors in clinical practice: a systematic review. Breast Cancer Res Treat. 2012;134(2):459–78.
84. Huiart L, Bouhnik A-D, Rey D, Tarpin C, Cluze C, Bendiane MK, et al. Early discontinuation of tamoxifen intake in younger women with breast cancer: is it time to rethink the way it is prescribed? Eur J Cancer Oxf Engl 1990. 2012;48(13):1939–46.
85. Sgroi DC, Sestak I, Cuzick J, Zhang Y, Schnabel CA, Schroeder B, et al. Prediction of late distant recurrence in patients with oestrogen-receptor-positive breast cancer: a prospective comparison of the breast-cancer index (BCI) assay, 21-gene recurrence score, and IHC4 in the TransATAC study population. Lancet Oncol. 2013;14(11):1067–76.
86. Dubsky P, Brase JC, Jakesz R, Rudas M, Singer CF, Greil R, et al. The EndoPredict score provides prognostic information on late distant metastases in ER+/HER2- breast cancer patients. Br J Cancer. 2013;109(12):2959–64.
87. Filipits M, Nielsen TO, Rudas M, Greil R, Stöger H, Jakesz R, et al. The PAM50 risk-of-recurrence score predicts risk for late distant recurrence after endocrine therapy in postmenopausal women with endocrine-responsive early breast cancer. Clin Cancer Res Off J Am Assoc Cancer Res. 2014;20(5):1298–305.
88. Swain SM, Jeong J-H, Geyer CE, Costantino JP, Pajon ER, Fehrenbacher L, et al. Longer therapy, iatrogenic amenorrhea, and survival in early breast cancer. N Engl J Med. 2010;362(22):2053–65.
89. Griggs JJ, Somerfield MR, Anderson H, Henry NL, Hudis CA, Khatcheressian JL, et al. American Society of Clinical Oncology endorsement of the cancer care Ontario practice guideline on adjuvant ovarian ablation in the treatment of premenopausal women with early-stage invasive breast cancer. J Clin Oncol Off J Am Soc Clin Oncol. 2011;29(29):3939–42.

90. Davidson NE, O'Neill AM, Vukov AM, Osborne CK, Martino S, White DR, et al. Chemoendocrine therapy for premenopausal women with axillary lymph node-positive, steroid hormone receptor-positive breast cancer: results from INT 0101 (E5188). J Clin Oncol Off J Am Soc Clin Oncol. 2005;23(25):5973–82.

91. International Breast Cancer Study Group (IBCSG), Castiglione-Gertsch M, O'Neill A, Price KN, Goldhirsch A, Coates AS, et al. Adjuvant chemotherapy followed by goserelin versus either modality alone for premenopausal lymph node-negative breast cancer: a randomized trial. J Natl Cancer Inst. 2003;95(24):1833–46.

92. Arriagada R, Lê MG, Spielmann M, Mauriac L, Bonneterre J, Namer M, et al. Randomized trial of adjuvant ovarian suppression in 926 premenopausal patients with early breast cancer treated with adjuvant chemotherapy. Ann Oncol Off J Eur Soc Med Oncol ESMO. 2005;16(3):389–96.

93. LHRH-Agonists in Early Breast Cancer Overview Group, Cuzick J, Ambroisine L, Davidson N, Jakesz R, Kaufmann M, et al. Use of luteinising-hormone-releasing hormone agonists as adjuvant treatment in premenopausal patients with hormone-receptor-positive breast cancer: a meta-analysis of individual patient data from randomised adjuvant trials. Lancet. 2007;369(9574):1711–23.

94. Gnant M, Mlineritsch B, Schippinger W, Luschin-Ebengreuth G, Pöstlberger S, Menzel C, et al. Endocrine therapy plus zoledronic acid in premenopausal breast cancer. N Engl J Med. 2009;360(7):679–91.

95. Pagani O, Regan MM, Walley BA, Fleming GF, Colleoni M, Láng I, et al. Adjuvant exemestane with ovarian suppression in premenopausal breast cancer. N Engl J Med. 2014;371(2):107–18.

96. Gnant M, Mlineritsch B, Stoeger H, Luschin-Ebengreuth G, Heck D, Menzel C, et al. Adjuvant endocrine therapy plus zoledronic acid in premenopausal women with early-stage breast cancer: 62-month follow-up from the ABCSG-12 randomised trial. Lancet Oncol. 2011;12(7):631–41.

97. Tevaarwerk AJ, Wang M, Zhao F, Fetting JH, Cella D, Wagner LI, et al. Phase III comparison of tamoxifen versus tamoxifen plus ovarian function suppression in premenopausal women with node-negative, hormone receptor-positive breast cancer (E-3193, INT-0142): a trial of the Eastern Cooperative Oncology Group. J Clin Oncol 2014;32(35):3948–58.

98. Francis PA, Regan MM, Fleming GF, Lang I, Ciruelos E, Bellet M, et al. Adjuvant ovarian suppression in premenopausal breast cancer. N Engl J Med 2015;375(5):436–46.

99. Pfeiler G, Königsberg R, Fesl C, Mlineritsch B, Stoeger H, Singer CF, et al. Impact of body mass index on the efficacy of endocrine therapy in premenopausal patients with breast cancer: an analysis of the prospective ABCSG-12 trial. J Clin Oncol Off J Am Soc Clin Oncol. 2011;29(19):2653–9.

100. Huober J, von Minckwitz G, Denkert C, Tesch H, Weiss E, Zahm DM, et al. Effect of neoadjuvant anthracycline-taxane-based chemotherapy in different biological breast cancer phenotypes: overall results from the GeparTrio study. Breast Cancer Res Treat. 2010;124(1): 133–40.

101. Loibl S. Neoadjuvant chemotherapy in the very young, 35 years of age or younger. SABCS. 2012; Abstract S3-1.

102. Masuda N, Sagara Y, Kinoshita T, Iwata H, Nakamura S, Yanagita Y, et al. Neoadjuvant anastrozole versus tamoxifen in patients receiving goserelin for premenopausal breast cancer (STAGE): a double-blind, randomised phase 3 trial. Lancet Oncol. 2012;13(4):345–52.

103. Torrisi R, Bagnardi V, Pruneri G, Ghisini R, Bottiglieri L, Magni E, et al. Antitumour and biological effects of letrozole and GnRH analogue as primary therapy in premenopausal women with ER and PgR positive locally advanced operable breast cancer. Br J Cancer. 2007;97(6):802–8.

104. Torrisi R, Bagnardi V, Rotmensz N, Scarano E, Iorfida M, Veronesi P, et al. Letrozole plus GnRH analogue as preoperative and adjuvant therapy in premenopausal women with ER positive locally advanced breast cancer. Breast Cancer Res Treat. 2011;126(2):431–41.

105. Cardoso F, Costa A, Norton L, Senkus E, Aapro M, André F, et al. ESO-ESMO 2nd international consensus guidelines for advanced breast cancer (ABC2). Breast Edinb Scotl. 2014;23(5):489–502.
106. Cardoso F, Loibl S, Pagani O, Graziottin A, Panizza P, Martincich L, et al. The European Society of Breast Cancer Specialists recommendations for the management of young women with breast cancer. Eur J Cancer Oxf Engl 1990. 2012;48(18):3355–77.
107. Klijn JG, Blamey RW, Boccardo F, Tominaga T, Duchateau L, Sylvester R, et al. Combined tamoxifen and luteinizing hormone-releasing hormone (LHRH) agonist versus LHRH agonist alone in premenopausal advanced breast cancer: a meta-analysis of four randomized trials. J Clin Oncol Off J Am Soc Clin Oncol. 2001;19(2):343–53.
108. Roché H. Anastrozole and goserelin combination as first treatment for premenopausal receptor positive advanced or metastatic breast cancer: a phase II trial. J Clin Oncol. 2009(2715s Suppl; Abstr 1079).
109. Nishimura R. Anastrozole and goserelin combination as first treatment for premenopausal receptor positive advanced or metastatic breast cancer: a phase II trial. J Clin Oncol. 2012(30 Suppl; Abstr 588).
110. Forward DP, Cheung KL, Jackson L, Robertson JFR. Clinical and endocrine data for goserelin plus anastrozole as second-line endocrine therapy for premenopausal advanced breast cancer. Br J Cancer. 2004;90(3):590–4.
111. Carlson RW, Theriault R, Schurman CM, Rivera E, Chung CT, Phan S-C, et al. Phase II trial of anastrozole plus goserelin in the treatment of hormone receptor-positive, metastatic carcinoma of the breast in premenopausal women. J Clin Oncol Off J Am Soc Clin Oncol. 2010;28(25):3917–21.
112. Park IH, Ro J, Lee KS, Kim E-A, Kwon Y, Nam B-H, et al. Phase II parallel group study showing comparable efficacy between premenopausal metastatic breast cancer patients treated with letrozole plus goserelin and postmenopausal patients treated with letrozole alone as first-line hormone therapy. J Clin Oncol Off J Am Soc Clin Oncol. 2010;28(16):2705–11.
113. Yao S, Xu B, Li Q, Zhang P, Yuan P, Wang J, et al. Goserelin plus letrozole as first- or second-line hormonal treatment in premenopausal patients with advanced breast cancer. Endocr J. 2011;58(6):509–16.
114. Cheung KL, Agrawal A, Folkerd E, Dowsett M, Robertson JFR, Winterbottom L. Suppression of ovarian function in combination with an aromatase inhibitor as treatment for advanced breast cancer in pre-menopausal women. Eur J Cancer Oxf Engl 1990. 2010;46(16):2936–42.
115. Bartsch R, Bago-Horvath Z, Berghoff A, DeVries C, Pluschnig U, Dubsky P, et al. Ovarian function suppression and fulvestrant as endocrine therapy in premenopausal women with metastatic breast cancer. Eur J Cancer Oxf Engl 1990. 2012;48(13):1932–8.

Impact of Breast Cancer Treatment on Fertility

3

Lorenzo Rossi and Olivia Pagani

3.1 Introduction

Despite breast cancer (BC) is a disease of postmenopausal women (the incidence gradually increases from 0.1/100,000 for women <20 years to 100–350/100,000 for women ≥70 years [1]), approximately 7 % of cases in the developed world and 25 % of patients in the developing world [2] are diagnosed in young women (i.e., <40 years). BC accounts for >40 % of all cancers in this age group (Table 3.1) and recent data show BC incidence in young women is increasing [3].

Young age, even after adjustment for socio-demographic and tumor characteristics, is generally considered an independent predictor of poorer survival after BC [4]. In a series of 873 patients aged ≤45 years from 20 public data sets, proliferation gene signatures showed no significant interaction with age in estrogen receptor positive/human epidermal growth factor receptor negative (ER+/HER2−) tumors but an inferior relapse-free survival was suggested in this subgroup as compared to women >40 years at diagnosis [2]. On the contrary, the outcome of 315 very young patients (<35 years at BC diagnosis) with Luminal A subtype who received adjuvant endocrine therapy (ET) was similar to that of older women [5].

The increased number of long-term young BC survivors has focused the attention of healthcare professionals to long-term adverse effects of cancer therapies. In addition to the risk of heart failure and secondary neoplasms, oncologists must consider the impact of antineoplastic treatments on premature ovarian failure and, thus, on fertility.

Young women with BC often face dilemmas about fertility, pregnancy, breastfeeding, and contraception. In the last decades, a trend toward delaying childbearing has been observed and the number of childless women at BC diagnosis is still likely to

L. Rossi • O. Pagani (✉)
Oncology Institute of Southern Switzerland (IOSI), Ospedale San Giovanni,
via Ospedale, Bellinzona 6500, Switzerland
e-mail: Lorenzo.Rossi@eoc.ch; Olivia.Pagani@eoc.ch

© Springer International Publishing Switzerland 2015   29
N. Biglia, F.A. Peccatori (eds.), *Breast Cancer, Fertility Preservation
and Reproduction*, DOI 10.1007/978-3-319-17278-1_3

Table 3.1 Incidence of breast cancer by age

Age	Annual incidence
<20	0.1/100,000
20–24	1.4/100,000
25–29	8.1/100,000
30–34	24.8/100,000
35–39	58.4/100,000
40–44	116.1/100,000

Modified by Pagani and Goldhirsh (2000) [6]

increase. A significant number of premenopausal BC survivors in the USA (approximately 20,000 women) were estimated to be at risk for infertility [7], and about half of them might want children and could benefit from fertility counseling and preservation. Preliminary data of the Helping Ourselves, Helping Others (HOHO) study, a prospective observational study conducted in the USA in women with BC diagnosed <40 years to address disease and psychosocial outcomes at diagnosis and during long-term (10 years) follow-up, show that 68 % of women discussed fertility issues with their physicians before starting therapy and 51 % were concerned about becoming infertile after treatment [8]. Despite these worries, only 10 % of patients took special steps to lessen the chance of infertility. Eleven percent of the studied population also considered receiving ET for <5 years. Unpublished preliminary data from the cohort of women followed outside the USA, within the International Breast Cancer Group (IBCSG) HOHO study (IBCSG 43–09), show that 20 % of patients desire children after BC and are willing to take <5 years of adjuvant tamoxifen. A prospective survey in 212 evaluable patients with ER+ early BC, less than 37 years at diagnosis, from 5 regions (Europe/US/Canada/Middle-East/Australia) showed almost 40% of patients were interested in a study of ET interruption to allow pregnancy [9].

The impact of anticancer treatments on reproductive organs may be direct (e.g., pelvic surgery or irradiation) or by influence of the hormonal milieu (e.g., ET, chemotherapy, targeted therapies, alteration of the pituitary axis subsequent to cranial irradiation).

3.2 Cytotoxic Chemotherapy and Targeted Therapies

Ovaries contain a fixed pool of oocytes that do not proliferate and are not replaced and whose number declines with age. Cytotoxic chemotherapy affects primordial follicles, oocytes, and granulosa cells. The most relevant toxic effect is the loss of follicles under maturation which results in ovulatory dysfunction and subsequent amenorrhea. Follicular atrophy can be reversed according to the number of active follicles remaining after the end of chemotherapy. As a consequence, the probability of chemotherapy-induced amenorrhea (CIA) depends on the age at the time of treatment, the type of chemotherapy received, its duration, and drug/s cumulative doses. Overall, the rate of CIA is between 20 % and 70 % in women <40 years but can approach 100 % in women >40 years (Table 3.2).

Table 3.2 Risk of chemotherapy-induced amenorrhea

Age	Regimen	Degree of risk
<30	AC×4 and docetaxel×4	6 %
	CMF, CEF, or CAF×6	<20 %
30–39	AC×4 and docetaxel×4	12 %
	AC, EC×4	<20 %
	CMF, CEF, or CAF×6	30–70 %
≥40	AC×4 and docetaxel×4	35 %
	AC, EC×4	30–70 %
	CMF, CEF, or CAF×6	>80 %
All age	Methotrexate+fluorouracil	Very low
	Monoclonal antibodies	Little evidence
	Taxanes	Little evidence

AC doxorubicin, cyclophosphamide, *CAF* cyclophosphamide, doxorubicin, fluorouracil, *CEF* cyclophosphamide, epirubicin, fluorouracil, *CMF* cyclophosphamide, Methotrexate, fluorouracil, *EC* epirubicin, cyclophosphamide

The two main mechanisms of chemotherapy-induced ovarian toxicity are direct follicle and oocyte apoptosis [10] and vascular damage [11]. Compared to untreated women, patients having received chemotherapy show a significantly lower follicle count [10]. Another important mechanism of ovarian injury is focal damage of the ovarian cortex through hyalinization of cortical vessels and intimal fibrosis. Ovaries exposed to chemotherapy show several areas of focal cortical subcapsular fibrosis [12].

CIA can either be "temporary" or "permanent." Temporary amenorrhea is mainly related to insufficient follicle development and alteration of hypothalamic function by disrupted estrogen metabolism. Permanent amenorrhea is more closely related to the direct toxicity of chemotherapy on the ovarian reserve. Transient menstrual irregularity or amenorrhea is common during chemotherapy, but a proportion of patients will resume menses within 6–12 months from treatment completion [13], the time required for damaged developing follicles to be replaced by new follicles from the remaining primordial follicle pool.

The most frequently used drugs in BC are alkylating agents (cyclophosphamide), anthracyclines, taxanes, and antimetabolites (methotrexate, 5-fluorouracil, capecitabine, gemcitabine). Alkylating agents are associated with the highest ovarian toxicity. The median dose of cyclophosphamide required to induce amenorrhea increases with decreasing age (5 g in 40-year-old patients, 9 g in 30-year-old patients, 20.4 g in patients <30 years). No data are available on the incidence of amenorrhea after single-agent anthracyclines. On the contrary, the anthracycline-containing combination regimens are highly toxic on ovarian function: about 34 % of women receiving the AC regimen (doxorubicin+cyclophosphamide) develop amenorrhea; CEF (cyclophosphamide-epirubicin-5-fluorouracil) and CMF (cyclophosphamide-methotrexate-5-fluorouracil) are associated with greater ovarian toxicity, with reported amenorrhea rates of 51 % and 43 %, respectively. The impact of taxanes on primordial follicles is still unclear. The addition of paclitaxel to the AC regimen, concurrently or sequentially, does not apparently increase the rate of amenorrhea [14]. Antimetabolites are less toxic for ovaries [15].

Fertility can be compromised even if women continue or resume menses after chemotherapy [16], and they can undergo early menopause due to the loss of a significant proportion of their primordial follicle pool [17]. Anthracycline- and/or cyclophosphamide-containing regimens may determine a loss of ovarian reserve of about 10 years, i.e., the amount of primordial follicles of women aged 26–27 years after this type of combination chemotherapy is similar to that of women aged 36–37 years. The reduction in the antimüllerian hormone (AMH), the best biochemical marker of ovarian reserve currently available, was shown to be associated with a loss of ovarian reserve of about 10 years [18]. Low pretreatment AMH was also found to be an independent predictor of CIA at 2 years after the end of chemotherapy ($P=0.005$; odds ratio 0.013), independently from age, in 59 premenopausal women with early BC, as compared with other markers of ovarian function (FSH and inhibin B) [19].

Patients with triple-negative BCs and BRCA mutation carriers often have multiple deficits in DNA repair pathways and may selectively benefit from platinum derivatives and Poly-(ADP-ribose) polymerase (PARP) inhibitors [20]. Trials are ongoing, but PARP inhibitors are likely to be less gonadotoxic than cyclophosphamide-based regimens. In a study of 168 cancer patients (38 with BC), the odds ratio (OR) of platinum-related ovarian failure in exposed versus unexposed patients was 1.77, second only to alkylating agents (OR 3.98) [21]. The available data with trastuzumab [16] report no increase in the likelihood of CIA. Data on bevacizumab are limited to patients with colorectal cancer: ovarian failure occurred in 34 % of women receiving a bevacizumab-containing regimen compared with 2 % of women receiving the same regimen without bevacizumab. Only approximately one fifth of these women recovered ovarian function and the US Food and Drug Administration (FDA) issued a warning in 2011 in order to properly inform women before starting treatment [22]. Information with newer chemotherapy agents or other targeted drugs (e.g., epothilones, lapatinib, pertuzumab) is missing.

A recent meta-analysis of 15,916 premenopausal BC patients from 46 studies showed that cyclophosphamide- taxane- and anthracyclines-based regimens significantly increased the incidence of CIA with pooled ORs of 2.25 (95 % CI 1.26–4.03, $p=0.006$), 1.26 (95 % CI 1.11–1.43, $p=0.0003$), and 1.39 (95 % CI 1.15–1.70, $p=0.0008$), respectively. The three-drug combination regimens of cyclophosphamide, anthracyclines, and taxanes caused the highest rate of CIA compared with other three-drug combinations (OR 1.41, 95 % CI 1.16–1.73, $P=0.0008$). The addition of tamoxifen was also associated with a higher incidence of CIA, with an OR of 1.48 [23].

The impact of cytotoxic therapy on ovarian function and fertility possibly depends not only on the type of drug and its cumulative doses, but also on the type of schedule chosen. It is well known that for some drugs (i.e., paclitaxel) the use of different schedules is correlated with variations of their pharmacodynamics [24]. It is therefore intuitive to think that a metronomic administration (often used in the metastatic setting) may be less toxic on the ovary, despite no data to confirm this hypothesis.

3.3   Endocrine Therapy

Being estrogen promoters, and possibly initiators, of most BCs, blocking their synthesis/function represents a logic therapeutic target in women with ER+ BC. In premenopausal women estrogen synthesis primarily occurs in the ovaries, but also in fat tissue, muscles, skin, stromal breast cells, adrenal glands, and in the neoplastic tissue itself.

The most commonly prescribed endocrine pharmacological treatments are selective estrogen receptor modulators (SERMs) (i.e., tamoxifen and toremifen), gonadotropin-releasing-hormone agonists (GnRHa), and aromatase inhibitors (AIs). In premenopausal women, tamoxifen for at least 5 years is a standard of care [25].

GnRHa have been introduced in the treatment of BC in premenopausal women at the end of the 1980s. GnRHa have a biphasic effect on the pituitary gland. Initially, they stimulate the secretion of both follicle-stimulating-(FSH) and luteinizing hormone (LH), while with long-term continuous administration, pituitary cells become resistant. The final result is a reversible inhibition of FSH and LH secretion and a fall in circulating levels of sex hormones similar to that produced by irreversible surgical- or radiation-induced castration. Serum levels of 17 beta-estradiol and progesterone fall within the 3rd–4th week after therapy start and the levels of LH and FSH remain suppressed. If a GnRHa is given, estradiol levels should be checked on a regular basis (at least every 6 months) because in some patients ovarian suppression is not achieved [26].

The recently published results of the Suppression of Ovarian Function Trial (SOFT) showed that, after a median follow-up of 67 months, the addition of ovarian function suppression/ablation (OFS/OA) to tamoxifen did not result in a significant benefit in terms of disease-free-survival (DFS) in the overall study population. However, for women who were considered at sufficient risk for recurrence to warrant adjuvant chemotherapy and who remained premenopausal after a median of 8 months after its completion, the addition of OFS significantly improved disease outcomes, especially if younger than 35 years at diagnosis [27].

Recent data from the randomized trials Tamoxifen and Exemestane Trial (TEXT) and SOFT also showed that the AI exemestane plus OFS/OA significantly reduces recurrences as compared with tamoxifen plus OFS/OA [28]. On the other hand, the ATLAS and aTToM trials represent the first evidence of a beneficial effect of extended adjuvant tamoxifen (10 years) in premenopausal women [29, 30]. As a consequence of these data supporting complete estrogen deprivation and/or longer duration of ET, larger numbers of women will be older and thus at higher risk for infertility at the time their therapy is completed.

Oophorectomy remains a viable ovarian suppression option both in the adjuvant and metastatic setting. Ovarian ablation by radiation therapy (RT) (15–20 Gy in 10–18 fractions to a modified pelvic treatment volume) is generally as effective as surgical oophorectomy or GnRHa administration but may take some months to be complete [31, 32]. These last two techniques, which are associated with permanent ovarian suppression, might be more indicated in older premenopausal patients and represent a valid alternative especially in country with limited resources [33].

The impact of single-agent tamoxifen on ovarian function is not well understood, since the number of premenopausal patients not receiving also adjuvant chemotherapy in the literature is very small. Tamoxifen may interfere with normal negative pituitary feedback mechanisms resulting in increased secretion of gonadotropins and, hence, in increased ovarian estrogen production [34]. The consequent hyper-estrogenism can be associated with ovarian cysts and oligo-amenorrhea [35, 36]. Overall, the incidence of tamoxifen-induced amenorrhea ranges between 16 and 38 % [37]. Amenorrhea while on tamoxifen did not, in itself, translate in definitive menopause in 65 patients receiving single-agent adjuvant tamoxifen as compared to 68 patients treated with tamoxifen after adjuvant chemotherapy [38]. Women should therefore be informed of the possibility of getting pregnant while on tamoxifen, despite having amenorrhea, and of the need for adequate non-hormonal contraception [26].

As compared to permanent CIA, tamoxifen-induced oligo-amenorrhea and OFS induced by GnRHa are reversible and ovarian function usually recovers after 3–6 months from their discontinuation, as the ovarian reserve is not permanently damaged. This can avoid the burden of premature menopause and be particularly appealing in women who did not complete their childbearing before BC diagnosis. Within the Breast International Group (BIG)-North American Breast Cancer Group (NABCG) collaboration the IBCSG has just launched a trial (*Pregnancy Outcome and Safety of Interrupting Therapy for women with endocrine responsIVE* breast cancer – POSITIVE – IBCSG 48–14 – clintrials.gov NCT02308085) which will assess the pattern of fertility recovery and pregnancy in women with maternity desire under different ETs.

AIs interfere with the enzyme aromatase, which, in highly estrogen-sensitive tissues, such as the breast, uterus, vagina, bone, brain, heart, and blood vessels, is responsible for the final step of estrogen synthesis from androgens (androstenedione and testosterone). Premenopausal women have a large amount of aromatase substrate in the ovary: AIs induce, by a pituitary loop effect, a dramatic increase of gonadotrophins and a subsequent increase in hormone levels. AIs should therefore not be given to premenopausal women without the addition of a GnRHa. The initial surge in FSH and LH induced by GnRHa before pituitary suppression together with the ovarian stimulation triggered by AIs are also used for embryo/oocyte cryopreservation. Women should be counseled to use non-hormonal contraception both during the first weeks of treatment and afterwards as sustained ovarian suppression is not achieved in some patients. The preliminary results of the SOFT-EST prospective substudy, measuring serial serum estrogens in 116 patients under ET (either Tamoxifen or Exemestane) and GnRHa in the SOFT trial show that about 20 % of patients had suboptimal estrogen suppression [39].

3.4 Radiation Therapy

RT is recommended to all women who underwent conservative breast surgery because significantly reduces the rate of local recurrence and improves overall survival [40]. A boost on the tumor bed is of particular benefit in young women [41].

RT is also recommended to women who underwent mastectomy and have a high risk of loco-regional relapse [42].

Ovarian follicles are sensible to radiation damage. Adjuvant loco-regional RT for early BC is not associated with significant ovarian toxicity, although internal scatter radiation can reach the pelvis and ovaries (2.1–7.6 Gy). In the palliative setting, it is sometimes necessary to irradiate the pelvis, for the treatment of bone or visceral metastases. The dose tolerance of the ovary is dependent on several factors (the volume irradiated, the total radiation dose, the fractionation schedule, and the patient's age at the time of treatment). Radiation doses to the pelvis exceeding 24 Gy will likely produce permanent ovarian ablation, but lower doses can be associated with premature ovarian failure with increasing age [43]. Cranial irradiation, affecting the hypothalamic-pituitary axis, may also impair fertility [44].

3.5 Surgical Treatment

Breast surgery does not have an impact on fertility, except for oophorectomy, mainly performed in developing countries as a substitute of costly GnRHa therapy, or as prophylactic surgery in patients harboring BRCA1/2 mutations.

3.6 Fertility Assessment After Breast Cancer Treatment

When assessing the impact of different chemotherapies on fertility, many clinical trials used amenorrhea or menstrual irregularities, which are not reliable markers of infertility, as endpoints. Despite maintenance or resumption of regular menses after BC treatment, fertility may be compromised due to the poor quality of surviving oocytes [45]. Women with decreased ovarian reserve often have shorter, more regular cycles due to accelerated follicle development. Permanent amenorrhea is also not uniformly defined across studies. The most used definitions range from irregular menses in the 1st year after treatment completion to continuous cessation of menses for more than 1 year [46].

Ovarian function recovery (OFR) can be measured by monitoring circulating levels of FSH, LH, estradiol, inhibin B, and AMH. Decline in the ovarian reserve leads to low levels of estradiol, inhibin B, and AMH, normally produced by the granulosa cells of the ovarian follicles. AMH is the most sensitive of all these tests, as it is consistent throughout the menstrual cycle and more closely approximates the number of ovarian primordial follicles [47]. Low pre-chemotherapy AMH and older age were both statistically significant predictors of CIA ($p=0.04$ and $p=0.008$, respectively) in 124 patients with early BC participating in the multicenter randomized controlled trial ECOG5103 (doxorubicin-cyclophosphamide followed by paclitaxel with either placebo or one of two durations of bevacizumab therapy) [48].

The widespread use of hormone level's monitoring has been limited by costs, lack of sensitivity, and cross reproducibility of available assays. Single measurements reflect ovarian function only at that specific time point and therefore do not predict the potential for sustained ovarian recovery. In addition, the validity of these tests following chemotherapy for BC is not yet been validated, and not all authors agree on their reliability in this particular setting of patients. A new highly sensitive AMH assay, prospectively used and validated in a cohort of 98 women with early BC, showed a tenfold increased sensitivity as compared to AMH, inhibin B, FSH, and estradiol measured with standard methods. In particular, the study showed that, even in women with regular menses, AMH measured 2 years after chemotherapy was generally very low for their age (mean age 35 years) and similar to older women who did not receive chemotherapy (mean age 45 years) [49].

In addition to AMH, an ultrasound-guided estimation of ovarian volume and antral follicle count, a simple and relatively inexpensive technique [50], can be used to estimate ovarian reserve. The sensitivity and specificity of this method are still being evaluated.

3.7   Psychosocial Impact of Fertility Impairment

The impact of cancer-related infertility on long-term distress and quality of life (QoL) has been poorly investigated in BC patients.

In the above mentioned prospective HOHO study, 37 % of patients wished future biologic children before BC diagnosis as compared to 26 % at the time of survey and 9 % did not want more children because they were afraid that pregnancy would increase their risk of recurrence [8]. A cross-sectional survey was conducted by phone interview in 240 US young women (mean age at the time of survey 43.7 years) diagnosed with cancer (130 with BC), unselected for their desire for children at diagnosis, 5–10 years post-treatment. A significant higher distress, more intrusive thoughts, and avoidance strategies were experienced by childless women as compared to women with adopted/stepchildren and women with at least one biological child, irrespective of cancer type [51].

One-hundred and thirty-one women with early BC diagnosed ≤40 years, originally participating in the Women's Healthy Eating and Living (WHEL) Study evaluating the influence of diet on BC outcome, participated in the WHEL Survivorship Study to investigate whether the level of reproductive concerns after treatment was associated with long-term depressive symptoms. Data were collected an average of 12 years post-diagnosis: reproductive concerns were a significant contributor to persistent depressive symptoms ($p = 0.0002$) as were not having children, being nulliparous at diagnosis and treatment-related ovarian damage (all with $p < 0.01$) [52].

Most of the available surveys are retrospective; nonetheless, their results are similar to those reported in a large, population-based study ($N = 2,818$) of non-cancer patients with unresolved infertility which showed significantly less satisfaction with life, more depressive symptoms, and decreased self-esteem than in women with no fertility problems [53].

Infertility can also impair sexual and relationship functioning, as shown in non-cancer women with a diagnosis of infertility [54].

Adoption, oocyte donors, or gestational carriers can be difficult to pursue by BC survivors. BC patients looking for adoption may face discrimination from national and international agencies, as well as from birth mothers. A survey conducted in the USA among 11 cancer organizations, 6 international adoption agencies, and 7 adoption specialists showed that most cancer organizations (except the Young Survival Coalition – YSC) had limited information on both potential barriers to adoption and legal and disclosure requirements [55]. Cancer survivors represented 0.5–10 % of the surveyed adoption agencies: 3 out of 6 agencies wanted to know about a previous cancer history, the remaining did not, particularly in case of early stages and after 2 years of disease-free survival.

Less than 10 % of cancer survivors consider using oocyte donors or gestational carriers to become parents [56]. High out-of-pocket costs and legal restrictions (i.e., domestic versus transnational surrogacy) may also limit third-party reproduction.

Women concerned about inherited cancer were more likely to consider pre-implantation genetic diagnosis (PGD) (i.e., creating embryos through in vitro fertilization and discarding those harboring a known mutation), than to undergo elective termination of an affected fetus. On the contrary, only 36 % of women with hereditary breast and ovarian syndromes, surveyed during a US national conference, considered to use PGD in a future conception [57].

3.8   BRCA Mutation Carriers

Women carrying a *BRCA1* mutation might be more prone to CIA as a consequence of occult primary ovarian insufficiency [58, 59]. In a multicenter survey of 1,426 young women with a *BRCA1* or *BRCA2* mutation treated with chemotherapy for early BC, the risk of long-term CIA was not greater than among women who did not carry a mutation [60].

Prophylactic surgery (i.e., bilateral mastectomy and/or salpingo-oophorectomy) is often discussed as part of BC treatment planning in women with known BRCA mutations. Hysterectomy is not always performed in these patients leaving the theoretical possibility to deliver. Some studies [61] revealed no association between BC risk and exposure to fertility drugs in women with BRCA mutation but data are controversial.

Mutation testing is feasible by embryo biopsy and PGD and embryo selection after genetic testing is available in some countries [62]. A qualitative study of patient preferences in 33 BRCA1/2 US mutation carriers undergoing genetic counselling showed the majority of participants preferred to be informed of the availability of PGD but also deferred detailed discussion [63]. In a similar survey conducted in 77 Spanish individuals, 61 % considered ethical to offer PDG, 55 % would contemplate prenatal diagnosis (PND), 48 % PGD, and 30 % adoption [64]. Individuals >40 years and those with a diagnosis of malignancy were more likely to consider PGD. Most healthcare professionals were also in favor of discussing PND and PGD in subjects with hereditary cancer susceptibility.

3.9   Contraception After Breast Cancer

Pregnancy should be avoided during active treatment of BC. Both cytotoxic agents and ETs (e.g., tamoxifen) are highly toxic to the embryo and affect embryonic development. Tamoxifen-related amenorrhea is not always associated with ovarian failure but can hide the presence of hyperactive ovaries due to a positive feedback mechanism [35]. If the combination of oral ET and GnRHa is given, estradiol levels should be checked on a regular basis (at least every 6 months) because in some patients ovarian suppression is not achieved [37–39].

As a consequence, patients should be informed to undertake effective non-hormonal contraception while on treatment. For women not wishing future pregnancies sterilization is the safest contraceptive method, being failure rates <1 %. A number of minimally invasive surgical options for sterilization are available, including laparoscopic tubal ligation and hysteroscopic sterilization. Non-hormonal methods including intrauterine devices (copper IUD or coil) and barrier methods (condoms, cervical diaphragm) can be prescribed being aware that, even with perfect use, they are associated with a 15 % failure rate.

The use of hormonal contraceptives is generally discouraged [65], particularly in women with ER+ BC. The levonorgestrel-releasing (LNG) IUD (Mirena®) releases a controlled local high-dose and low systemic dose of progestins (52 mg). Local progestin therapy may be helpful in managing endometrial proliferation on tamoxifen, anemia, menorrhagia, and dysmenorrhea, especially in women with ER tumors. Population-based data show no increased risk of BC in women with LNG-IUD at BC diagnosis as compared to Cu-IUD users in 5,100 BC patients and 20,000 controls [66]. Studies in BC survivors are small [65]: a recent retrospective cohort study [67] compared 79 Belgian BC patients who used the LNG-IUD at diagnosis with a control group of 120 patients with no history of LNG-IUD use, closely matched for age, tumor characteristics, and treatment modalities. Overall, no increased risk of BC recurrence in patients with use of the LNG-IUD at diagnosis was reported, but a subgroup analysis showed a trend towards an increased recurrence rate in women who continued to use the LNG-IUD after diagnosis. Patients should be informed about the lack of safety data of LNG-IUD, and alternative contraception methods should be counselled.

The newer low-dose LNG-IUD (13.5 mg) (Skyla®) is effective, reversible, and associated with less anemia, menorrhagia, and dysmenorrhea compared to Cu-IUD. However, there is currently no evidence regarding its safety in the setting of BC [68].

The World Health Organization (WHO) guidelines do not identify medical conditions for which the risks of emergency contraception outweigh its benefits [70], and this method should therefore be available also to women diagnosed with and/or under treatment for BC. The prescribed emergency method should be tailored according to the time elapsed after the unprotected intercourse but should also take into account body mass index (BMI) which is often elevated in BC patients under ET. A reduced efficacy of emergency contraception has in fact been reported in women with elevated BMI [71].

A recent meta-analysis of three case-control studies confirmed a significantly decreased ovarian cancer risk in BRCA1/2 mutation carriers associated with the use of combined oral contraceptives. On the contrary, data on the risk of BC are heterogeneous and results are inconsistent [72].

3.10   Fertility and Advanced Breast Cancer

Discussing infertility risk and fertility preservation in women with advanced breast cancer (ABC) is challenging and it may seem inappropriate [73]. Despite the lack of data, it is likely that issues surrounding fertility are also concerning young women with ABC [74] and the improved outcomes and long-term survival achieved with modern therapies warrant new approaches by healthcare professional community in this patients' population.

A pilot study assessing the safety of re-implanting cryopreserved ovarian tissue from advanced-stage BC showed no contamination by malignant cells [75]. Further evidence is required before ovarian tissue transplantation can be contemplated in these patients but breast oncologists should provide an opportunity to discuss the topic, handling the conversation carefully and sensitively.

Conclusions

The pattern of fertility impairment from anticancer treatments in premenopausal women with BC is heterogeneous and deserves individualized, tailored approaches. Several discriminants (age; prognosis; treatment type and duration; personal, familial, social, and religious beliefs) contribute to the approach of both patients and health professionals towards fertility preservation attitudes and discussions. The improved outcome of young BC patients requires new strategies and opens new frontiers (i.e., gestational surrogacy, fertility in ABC patients, prenatal and pre-implantation genetic diagnosis, cost evaluation and coverage) which can be best addressed when multidisciplinary teams include a broad range of expertise. Oncology/breast nurses, together fertility specialists with social workers and psycho-oncologists, may play an important role in facilitating these discussions [76]. Lack of knowledge and clinicians' prejudices should not prevent young patients with BC the best support in all the steps of their disease journey.

References

1. Hery C, Ferlay J, Boniol M, et al. Quantification of changes in breast cancer incidence and mortality since 1990 in 35 countries with Caucasian-majority populations. Ann Oncol. 2008;19:1187–94.
2. Azim Jr HA, Michiels S, Bedard PL, et al. Elucidating prognosis and biology of breast cancer arising in young women using gene expression profiling. Clin Cancer Res. 2012;18(5):1341–51.
3. Merlo DF, Ceppi M, Filiberti R, et al. Breast cancer incidence trends in European women aged 20–39 years at diagnosis. Breast Cancer Res Treat. 2012;134:363–70.

4. Copson E, Eccles E, Maishman T, et al. Prospective observational study of breast cancer treatment outcomes for UK women aged 18–40 years at diagnosis: the POSH study. J Natl Cancer Inst. 2013;105:978–88.
5. Cancello G, Maisonneuve P, Rotmensz N, et al. Prognosis and adjuvant treatment effects in selected breast cancer subtypes of very young women (\35 years) with operable breast cancer. Ann Oncol. 2010;21(10):1974–81.
6. Pagani O, Goldhirsch A. Breast cancer in young women: climbing for progress in care and knowledge. Womens Health (Lond Engl). 2006;2(5):717–32. doi:10.2217/17455057.2.5.717.
7. Trivers KF, Fink AK, Partridge AH, et al. Estimates of young breast cancer survivors at risk for infertility in the U.S. Oncologist. 2014;19(8):814–22.
8. Ruddy KJ, Gelber SI, Tamimi RM, et al. Prospective study of fertility concerns and preservation strategies in young women with breast cancer. J Clin Oncol. 2014;32(11):1151–6.
9. Pagani O, Ruggeri M, Manunta S et al. Pregnany after breast cancer: are young patients willing to partecipate in clinical studies? Breast. 2015;S0960-9776(15)00006-5.
10. Oktem O, Oktay K. Quantitative assessment of the impact of chemotherapy on ovarian follicle reserve and stromal function. Cancer. 2007;110:2222–9.
11. Meirow D, Dor J, Kaufman B, et al. Cortical fibrosis and blood-vessels damage in human ovaries exposed to chemotherapy. Potential mechanisms of ovarian injury. Hum Reprod. 2007;22: 1626–33.
12. Morgan S, Anderson RA, Gourley C, et al. How do chemotherapeutic agents damage the ovary? Hum Reprod Update. 2012;18:525–35.
13. Jung M, Shin H, Rha S, et al. The clinical outcome of chemotherapy-induced amenorrhea in premenopausal young patients with breast cancer with long-term follow-up. Ann Surg Oncol. 2010;17(12):3259–68.
14. Fornier MN, Modi S, Panageas KS, et al. Incidence of chemotherapy induced, long-term amenorrhea in patients with breast carcinoma age 40 years and younger after adjuvant anthracycline and taxane. Cancer. 2005;104:1575–9.
15. Minton SE, Munster PN. Chemotherapy-induced amenorrhea and fertility in women undergoing adjuvant treatment for breast cancer. Cancer Control. 2002;9(6):466–72.
16. Abusief ME, Missmer SA, Ginsburg ES, et al. The effects of paclitaxel, dose density, and trastuzumab on treatment-related amenorrhea in premenopausal women with breast cancer. Cancer. 2010;116(4):791–8.
17. Partridge A, Gelber S, Gelber RD, et al. Age of menopause among women who remain premenopausal following treatment for early breast cancer: long-term results from international breast cancer study group trials V and VI. EJC. 2007;43:1646–53.
18. Rodiguez Wallberg KA, Oktay K. Fertility preservation and pregnancy in women with and without BRCA mutation–positive breast cancer. Oncologist. 2012;17:1409–17.
19. Anderson RA, Rosendahl M, Kelsey TW, et al. Pretreatment anti-Müllerian hormone predicts for loss of ovarian function after chemotherapy for early breast cancer. Eur J Cancer. 2013;49(16):3404–11.
20. Oakman C, Viale G, Di Leo A. Management of triple negative breast cancer. Breast. 2010;19(5):312–21.
21. Meirow D, Nugent D. The effects of radiotherapy and chemotherapy on female reproduction. Hum Reprod Update. 2001;7(6):535–43.
22. National Cancer Institute: FDA approval for bevacizumab. http://www.cancer.gov/cancertopics/druginfo/fda-bevacizumab
23. Zhao J, Liu J, Chen K, et al. What lies behind chemotherapy-induced amenorrhea for breast cancer patients: a meta-analysis. Breast Cancer Res Treat. 2014;145(1):113–28.
24. Joerger M. Metabolism of the taxanes including nab-paclitaxel. Expert Opin Drug Metab Toxicol. 2014;14:1–12.
25. Burstein HJ, Temin S, Anderson H, et al. Adjuvant endocrine therapy for women with hormone receptor-positive breast cancer: American Society of Clinical Oncology clinical practice guideline focused update. J Clin Oncol. 2014;32(21):2255–69.
26. Partridge AH, Pagani O, Abulkhair O, et al. First international consensus guidelines for breast cancer in young women (BCY1). Breast. 2014;23(3):209–20.

27. Francis PA, Regan MM, Fleming GF, et al. Adjuvant ovarian suppression in premenopausal breast cancer. N Engl J Med. 2014. doi:10.1056/NEJMoa1412379.
28. Pagani O, Regan MM, Walley BA, et al. Adjuvant exemestane with ovarian suppression in premenopausal breast cancer. N Engl J Med. 2014;371(2):107–18.
29. Davies C, Pan H, Godwin J, et al. Long-term effects of continuing adjuvant tamoxifen to 10 years versus stopping at 5 years after diagnosis of oestrogen receptor-positive breast cancer: ATLAS, a randomised trial. Lancet. 2013;381:805–16.
30. Gray RG, Rea D, Handley K, et al. aTTom: Long-term effects of continuing adjuvant tamoxifen to 10 years versus stopping at 5 years in 6,953 women with early breast cancer. J Clin Oncol. 2013;31(suppl):abstr 5.
31. Hughes LL, Gray RJ, Solin LJ, et al. Eastern Cooperative Oncology Group; Southwest Oncology Group; Cancer and Leukemia Group B; North Central Cancer Treatment Group. Efficacy of radiotherapy for ovarian ablation: results of a breast intergroup study. Cancer. 2004;101(5):969–72.
32. McDonald Wade 3rd S, Hackney MH, et al. Ovarian suppression in the management of premenopausal breast cancer: methods and efficacy in adjuvant and metastatic settings. Oncology. 2008;75(3–4):192–202.
33. Bese NS, Iribas A, Dirican A, et al. Ovarian ablation by radiation therapy: is it still an option for the ablation of ovarian function in endocrine responsive premenopausal breast cancer patients? Breast. 2009;18(5):304–8.
34. Jordan VC, Fritz NF, Langan-Fahey S, et al. Alteration of endocrine parameters in premenopausal women with breast cancer during long-term adjuvant therapy with tamoxifen as the single agent. J Natl Cancer Inst. 1991;83:1488–9.
35. Mourits MJ, Devries EG, Ten Hoor KA, et al. Beware of amenorrhea during tamoxifen: it may be a wolf in sheep's clothing. J Clin Oncol. 2007;25:3787–8.
36. Goodwin PJ, Ennis M, Pritchard KI, et al. Risk of menopause during the first year after breast cancer diagnosis. J Clin Oncol. 1999;17:2365–70.
37. Petrek J, Naughton M, Case D, et al. Incidence, time course, and determinants of menstrual bleeding after breast cancer treatment: a prospective study. J Clin Oncol. 2006;24:1045–51.
38. Berliere M, Duhoux FP, Dalenc F, et al. Tamoxifen and ovarian function. PLoS One. 2013;8:e66616.
39. Bellet M, Gray KP, Francis PA et al. Estrogen levels in premenopausal (prem) patients (pts) with hormone-receptor positive (HR+) early breast cancer (BC) receiving adjuvant triptorelin (Trip) plus exemestane (E) or tamoxifen (T) in the SOFT trial: SOFT-EST substudy. J Clin Oncol. 2014; 32:5s(suppl; abstr 585)
40. Early Breast Cancer Trialists Collaborative Group (EBCTCG), Darby S, McGale P, Correa C, et al. Effect of radiotherapy after breast-conserving surgery on 10-year recurrence and 15-year breast cancer death: meta-analysis of individual patient data for 10,801 women in 17 randomised trials. Lancet. 2011;378(9804):1707–16.
41. Antonini N, Jones H, Horiot JC, et al. Effect of age and radiation dose on local control after breast conserving treatment: EORTC trial 22881–10882. Radiother Oncol. 2007;82(3):265–71.
42. Li Y, Moran MS, Huo Q, et al. Post-mastectomy radiotherapy for breast cancer patients with t1-t2 and 1–3 positive lymph nodes: a meta-analysis. PLoS One. 2013;8(12):e81765.
43. Stroud JS, Mutch D, Rader J, et al. Effects of cancer treatment on ovarian function. Fertil Steril. 2009;92(2):417–27.
44. Resetkova N, Hayashi M, Kolp LA, et al. Fertility preservation for prepubertal girls: update and current challenges. Curr Obstet Gynecol Rep. 2013;2(4):218–25.
45. Partridge A, Gelber S, Gelber RD, et al. Age of menopause among women who remain premenopausal following treatment for early breast cancer: long-term results from International Breast Cancer Study Group Trials V and VI. Eur J Cancer. 2007;43:1646–53.
46. Walshe JM, Denduluri N, Swain SM. Amenorrhea in premenopausal women after adjuvant chemotherapy for breast cancer. J Clin Oncol. 2006;24:5769–79.
47. Anderson RA, Cameron DA. Pretreatment serum anti-mullerian hormone predicts long-term ovarian function and bone mass after chemotherapy for early breast cancer. J Clin Endocrinol Metab. 2011;96:1336–43.

48. Ruddy KJ, O'Neill A, Miller KD, et al. Biomarker prediction of chemotherapy-related amenorrhea in premenopausal women with breast cancer participating in E5103. Breast Cancer Res Treat. 2014;144(3):591–7.
49. Chai J, Howie AF, Cameron DA, et al. A highly-sensitive anti-Müllerian hormone assay improves analysis of ovarian function following chemotherapy for early breast cancer. Eur J Cancer. 2014;50(14):2367–74.
50. Scheffer GJ, Broekmans FJ, Looman CW, et al. The number of antral follicles in normal women with proven fertility is the best reflection of reproductive age. Hum Reprod. 2003;18:700–6.
51. Canada AL, Schover LR. The psychosocial impact of interrupted childbearing in long-term female cancer survivors. Psychooncology. 2012;21(2):134–43.
52. Gorman JR, Malcarne VL, Roesch SC, et al. Depressive symptoms among young breast cancer survivors: the importance of reproductive concerns. Breast Cancer Res Treat. 2010;123(2):477–85.
53. Schwerdtfeger KL, Shreffler KM. Trauma of pregnancy loss and infertility for mothers and involuntarily childless women in the contemporary United States. J Loss Trauma. 2009;14(3):211–27.
54. Millheiser LS, Helmer AE, Quintero RB, et al. Is infertility a risk factor for female sexual dysfunction? A case-control study. Fertil Steril. 2010;94(6):2022–5.
55. Rosen A. Third-party reproduction and adoption in cancer patients. J Natl Cancer Inst Monogr. 2005;34:91–3.
56. Schover LR, Rybicki LA, Martin BA, et al. Having children after cancer: a pilot survey of survivors' attitudes and experiences. Cancer. 1999;86:697–709.
57. Quinn G, Vadaparampil S, Wilson C, et al. Attitudes of high-risk women toward preimplantation genetic diagnosis. Fertil Steril. 2009;91(6):2361–8.
58. Oktay K, Kim JY, Barad D, et al. Association of BRCA1 mutations with occult primary ovarian insufficiency: a possible explanation for the link between infertility and breast/ovarian cancer risks. J Clin Oncol. 2010;28:240–4.
59. Wang ET, Pisarska MD, Bresee C, et al. BRCA1 germline mutations may be associated with reduced ovarian reserve. Steril. 2014. pii: S0015-0282(14)2073-1.
60. Valentini A, Finch A, Lubinski J, et al. Chemotherapy-induced amenorrhea in patients with breast cancer with a BRCA1 or BRCA2 mutation. J Clin Oncol. 2013;31:3914–9.
61. Kotsopoulos J, Librach CL, Lubinski J, et al. Infertility, treatment of infertility, and the risk of breast cancer among women with BRCA1 and BRCA2 mutations: a case-control study. Cancer Causes Control. 2008;19(10):1111–9. doi:10.1007/s10552-008-9175-0. Epub 2008 May 29.
62. Noble R, Bahadur G, Iqbal M, et al. Pandora's box: ethics of PGD for inherited risk of late-onset disorders. Reprod Biomed Online. 2008;17 Suppl 3:55–60.
63. Hurley K, Rubin LR, Werner-Lin A, et al. Incorporating information regarding preimplantation genetic diagnosis into discussions concerning testing and risk management for BRCA1/2 mutations: a qualitative study of patient preferences. Cancer. 2012;118(24):6270–7.
64. Donnelly LS, Watson M, Moynihan C, et al. Reproductive decision-making in young female carriers of a BRCA mutation. Hum Reprod. 2013;28(4):1006–12.
65. Centers for Disease Control and Prevention (CDC). United States Medical Eligibility Criteria (US MEC) for contraceptive use, 2010. Cited 2013-12-16. http://www.cdc.gov/reproductive-health/unintendedpregnancy/usmec.htm
66. Dinger J, Bardenheuer K, Minh TD. Levonorgestrel-releasing and copper intrauterine devices and the risk of breast cancer. Contraception. 2011;83:211–7.
67. Schwarz EB, Hess R, Trussell J. Contraception for cancer survivors. J Gen Intern Med. 2009;24 Suppl 2:S401e6.
68. Trinh XB, Tjalma WAA, Makar AP, et al. Use of the levonorgestrel-releasing intrauterine system in breast cancer patients. Fertil Steril. 2008;90:17–22.
69. Casey PM, Faubion SS, MacLaughlin KL, et al. Caring for the breast cancer survivor's health and well-being. World J Clin Oncol. 2014;5(4):693–704.
70. World Health Organization. Medical Eligibility Criteria for contraceptive use. Cited 2013-12-16. Available from: http://whqlibdoc.who.int/publications/2004/9241562668.pdf.

71. Glasier AF, Cameron ST, Fine PM, et al. Ulipristal acetate versus levonorgestrel for emergency contraception: a randomised non-inferiority trial and meta-analysis. Lancet. 2010;375: 555–62.
72. Cibula D, Zikan M, Dusek L, et al. Oral contraceptives and risk of ovarian and breast cancers in BRCA mutation carriers: a meta-analysis. Expert Rev Anticancer Ther. 2011;11(8): 1197–207.
73. Nieman CL, Kazer R, Brannigan RE, et al. Cancer survivors and infertility: a review of a new problem and novel answers. J Support Oncol. 2006;4:171–8.
74. Debono DJ, Kohnke JM, Helft PR. Addressing fertility in patients with advanced cancer: how the quality oncology practice initiative standards and ASCO guidelines facilitate ethical communication. J Oncol Pract. 2009;5(6):298–300.
75. Luyckx V, Durant JF, Camboni A, et al. Is transplantation of cryopreserved ovarian tissue from patients with advanced-stage breast cancer safe? A pilot study. J Assist Reprod Genet. 2013;30(10):1289–99.
76. McNees P. Technology application to assist young survivors with fertility concerns. Semin Oncol Nurs. 2009;25(4):284–87.

Fertility Preservation, ART, and Breast Cancer

4

Alberto Revelli, Francesca Salvagno, Simona Casano, Luisa Delle Piane, and Chiara Benedetto

4.1 Introduction

Fertility preservation is a key issue for young women and girls at high risk of ovarian insufficiency because of the gonadotoxic therapies required to treat breast cancer (BC).

The assessment of infertility risk should be individualized for every patient and the strategy to preserve fecundity after cancer treatment must be carefully planned considering the patient's age, the type of cancer, the type of treatment, the time available for fertility preservation procedure, and the risk of ovarian metastasis.

A strict cooperation between fertility preservation specialists and oncologists is fundamental to optimize a fertility preservation program.

According to the American Society of Clinical Oncology (ASCO) guidelines for fertility preservation in cancer patients, oncologists should be prepared to discuss the implications of chemotherapy on fertility with their patients as early as possible during treatment planning, or alternatively they should refer patients to reproductive specialists to discuss the risk of iatrogenic ovarian failure and fertility preservation options [1].

Current strategies for fertility preservation in women affected by breast cancer include oocyte and embryo cryopreservation, while experimental techniques are ovarian tissue cryopreservation and the use of GnRH analogs to induce ovarian functional suppression (Table 4.1) [2].

A. Revelli (✉) • F. Salvagno • S. Casano • L. Delle Piane • C. Benedetto
Department of Surgical Sciences, University of Torino, Sant'Anna Hospital,
Via Ventimiglia 3, Torino 10126, Italy
e-mail: alberto.revelli@unito.it; francesca.salvagno@yahoo.it; simona.casano@libero.it;
l.dellepiane@iol.it; chiara.benedetto@unito.it

© Springer International Publishing Switzerland 2015   45
N. Biglia, F.A. Peccatori (eds.), *Breast Cancer, Fertility Preservation
and Reproduction*, DOI 10.1007/978-3-319-17278-1_4

Table 4.1 Fertility preservation options in BC patients

Fertility preservation options	Standard strategy	Ovarian stimulation required	Invasive procedure required	Male partner required	Risk of malignant cells contamination	Delay in cancer treatment	Available in all centers
Oocyte cryopreservation	+	+	+	–	–	+	–
Embryo cryopreservation	+	+	+	+	–	+	–
Ovarian suppression with GnRH analogs	–	–	–	–	–	–	+
Ovarian tissue cryopreservation	–	–	++	–	+	–	–

4.2   Mature Oocyte and Embryo Cryopreservation

Controlled ovarian hyperstimulation (COH) with gonadotropins is needed to obtain more than one oocyte and is a key component in the success of in vitro fertilization (IVF), as well as in cycles aiming to preserve fertility by oocyte or embryo cryostorage [3]. The choice of the specific COH protocol is generally based on the preferences of each IVF unit and is influenced by the time available before the initiation of radio-/chemotherapy. Although multiple different COH protocols have been proposed, the majority of patients are treated with a GnRH antagonist short protocol, which allows the shortest deferral of the initiation of chemotherapy [4].

Conventionally, ovarian stimulation with GnRH antagonists can be started either in the early follicular phase or in the luteal phase [4]. The first approach requires awaiting menses: gonadotropin stimulation begins on day 2–3 of the cycle, while GnRH antagonist is usually started on day 6, when the size of the leading follicle reaches 12–14 mm [5]. Administration of a GnRH antagonist (e.g., 3 mg cetrorelix subcutaneously) in the luteal phase, instead, induces corpus luteum breakdown and menstruation ensues a few days later [6, 7]. Ovarian stimulation can therefore be initiated quickly and the GnRH antagonist would be restarted later to prevent premature LH surge [7].

Recently, the introduction in the clinical practice of the so-called "random-start" ovarian stimulation protocol has provided a further decrease of the total time required for ovarian stimulation [4]. This novel technique is supported by the demonstration of a series of three major follicle-recruiting waves during a normal menstrual cycle, allowing to start follicular growth irrespective of the cycle phase [3]. In fact, in the "random-start" protocol, COH can be initiated either in the late follicular phase or in the luteal phase, following spontaneous LH surge or after ovulation induction with human chorionic gonadotrophin (hCG) or a GnRH agonist (Fig. 4.1) [3]. Both these ovarian stimulation strategies are as effective as conventional start protocols [8], challenging the traditional concept that antral follicles observed in the luteal phase have undergone atresia and are useless [8, 9].

During COH there is a potential risk that the supra-physiologic estradiol (E2) levels could promote the growth of estrogen receptor-positive (ER+) breast cancer cells [10]. The rise in E2 is directly proportional to the number of growing follicles; for this reason, alternative and potentially safer protocols have been introduced for these patients, including natural cycle IVF, stimulation protocols with tamoxifen (TAM) alone or combined with gonadotropins, and stimulation protocols with aromatase inhibitors (AI) [11].

Natural cycle IVF does not allow to obtain more than one oocyte or embryo per cycle and has a high rate of cycle cancellation due to precocious follicle rupture. This strategy may thus result ineffective when chemotherapy is imminent and the patient does not have a chance for a second attempt [11].

TAM is a non-steroidal compound related to clomiphene, as effective as clomiphene for COH in anovulatory patients [12]. TAM is a selective ER modulator (SERM) with antioestrogenic actions on breast tissue leading to inhibition of the growth of breast tumors due to competitive antagonism of E2 at its receptor site [12]. TAM can be used for ovulation induction starting on day 2–5 of the menstrual cycle in doses of 20–60 mg/day; it may be used alone or in combination with gonadotropins [13]. Ovulation

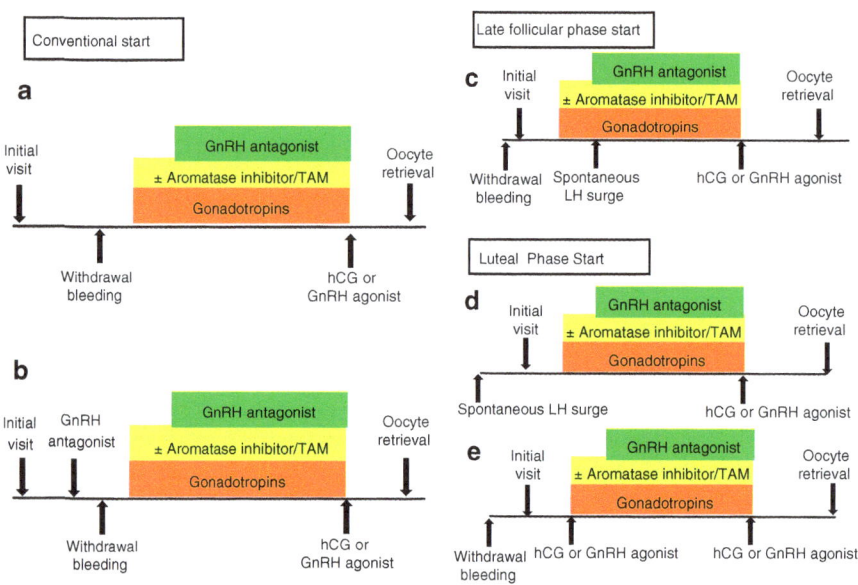

Fig. 4.1 Conventional and random-start COH. (**a**) Conventional start in early follicular phase, (**b**) conventional start in luteal phase after luteolysis induced by GnRH antagonist, (**c**) random start in late follicular phase, (**d**) random start in luteal phase following spontaneous LH surge or after ovulation induction with hCG or GnRH agonist (**e**)

induction with TAM for fertility preservation in cancer patients has been shown to increase mature oocyte and embryo yield compared with natural cycle IVF, reducing cycle cancellation rate [13]. The combination of low-dose FSH with TAM further increased the number of cryopreserved oocytes and embryos compared with ovulation induction with TAM alone [14]. Although E2 levels during COH with TAM are not very low, its use in ER+ breast cancer patients is protective, due to its antiestrogenic effect on breast tissue [13]. The safety of TAM coadministration during COH has been recently confirmed by the assessment of persistently high serum E2 levels in premenopausal breast cancer patients safely treated with adjuvant TAM, at up to 6 years follow-up [15].

AI, such as letrozole, markedly suppress plasma E2 levels by competitively inhibiting the activity of the enzyme aromatase [16]. Aromatase is a cytochrome P450 enzyme complex that catalyzes the conversion of androstenedione and testosterone to estrone and E2, respectively [17]. Centrally, AI release the hypothalamic-pituitary axis from the estrogenic negative feedback, increase the pituitary secretion of FSH, stimulate follicle growth, and, thereby, can be used for ovulation induction [18]. The use of letrozole alone for ovarian stimulation has been associated with lower E2 levels than those observed in a natural cycle [19]. Oktay tested letrozole in association with gonadotropins and a GnRH antagonist ("COST-LESS" protocol) [14]: letrozole was started orally from day 2 or 3 of the cycle at a dose of 5 mg day, while gonadotropins (150–300 UI) were started 2 days later. A GnRH antagonist was added when E2 levels exceeded 250 pg/ml or when the leading follicle reached 14 mm diameter in order to prevent premature LH surge. All medications were discontinued the day of hCG trigger, and letrozole was reinitiated after oocyte retrieval and continued until E2 levels fell to 550 pg/ml. The final maturity of oocytes was triggered with hCG, that, however, potentiates the endogenous production of E2 during the luteal phase, may cause ovarian hyperstimulation syndrome (OHSS) and can cause a false-positive pregnancy test, creating confusion when a pregnancy test is performed prior to initiation of chemotherapy [10]. In order to circumvent these problems, hCG trigger was later replaced by GnRH agonist trigger (1 mg leuprolide acetate), leading to significantly faster drop in E2 levels, significantly lower rate of moderate/severe OHSS and comparable number of mature oocytes [20]. Compared to a conventional IVF protocol, the COST-LESS protocol resulted in a significantly lower peak estradiol levels and in a 44 % reduction in gonadotropin requirement, while the length of stimulation, the number of embryos obtained, and the fertilization rate were similar [14].

Stimulation protocols using letrozole are currently preferred over TAM protocols for patients with ER+ breast cancer who need fertility preservation because it allows to minimize the risk of high E2 exposure [14] and of cancer recurrence [21].

Maximizing the number of embryos or oocytes cryopreserved during a fertility preservation cycle is extremely important to increase the chance of future pregnancies: cancer patients have shortage of time and often a single COH cycle to try [22]. Traditionally, breast cancer patients have time to undergo one cycle of COH before initiating adjuvant chemotherapy, which typically occurs after breast surgery [3]. In the event of a poor response, multiple cycles are often not feasible owing to time constraints. Unfortunately in cancer patients, both the specific malignancy and the patient's general conditions may have a negative impact on the response to ovarian stimulation [23]. In breast cancer, some authors [24] reported that in BRCA1 mutation-positive patients a low response to ovarian stimulation occurred significantly more frequently than in patients with BRCA2 or without BRCA mutation. BRCA genes play an essential role in double-strand DNA break repair, and their mutations are associated with an increased risk of breast and ovarian cancers [24]. In patients with BRCA mutations, oocytes may be more prone to DNA damage, clinically manifesting as diminished ovarian reserve, poor ovarian response to COH, or earlier menopause [25].

One of the most obvious strategies to increase the embryo and oocyte yield could be the use of higher doses of gonadotropins [3]; surprisingly, a recent evidence suggests that a high-dose FSH stimulation does not improve pregnancy outcomes, and may be associated with a lower live birth rate [26], supporting the theory that high doses of FSH might stimulate the recruitment of chromosomally abnormal or incompetent oocytes [27]. Another strategy to improve oocyte yield is the early referral (before breast surgery) that allows breast cancer patients to undergo multiple COH cycles without delaying the initiation of adjuvant chemotherapy [28].

4.3 Ovarian Tissue Cryopreservation

Ovarian tissue cryopreservation (OTC) is the main option available to preserve fertility in women under the age of 38 years who require urgent cancer treatments, such as neo-adjuvant chemotherapy. OTC does not need ovarian stimulation and is independent from menstrual cycle: it can be performed in a few days, without any delay in the beginning of chemotherapy.

OTC allows to retrieve and cryostore a great number of primordial follicles that are relatively resistant to cryodamage [29]. Moreover, this technique permits to restore endocrine function after reimplantation of ovarian tissue and is the only option for prepubertal patients. The main disadvantage of the strategy is the need of invasive procedures both for tissue harvesting and transplantation. Of note, OTC may cause a further decrease of ovarian reserve as an effect of ovarian surgery. Another crucial point is the risk of reintroducing malignant cells when transplantation is performed.

It has not yet been established whether ovarian biopsy or unilateral oophorectomy should be preferable to retrieve ovarian tissue. Indeed patients who underwent unilateral oophorectomy were reported to have a significant number of spontaneous pregnancies; however, the removal of an entire ovary might be too aggressive, and could reduce the ovarian reserve too much [30]. Several studies concluded that laparoscopy should be considered the gold standard for ovarian tissue harvesting, although ovarian tissue can be obtained during contingent laparotomic surgeries when these are needed [31]. When ovarian tissue has been recovered, transport on ice from the place of removal to the laboratory can last up to 20 h, thus allowing the creation of few specialized centers where cryopreservation procedure takes place [32]. In the laboratory ovarian cortex is enucleated from the medulla and cut in small fragments. One or two fragments are usually sent to histology. Ex vivo retrieval of mature or immature oocytes and their vitrification (after in vitro maturation in case of immature oocytes) is feasible and improves the efficiency of fertility preservation programs [33]. Finally the ovarian tissue is stored in liquid nitrogen after the freezing procedure. Although slow freezing of ovarian cortex is still applied in most fertility preservation laboratories and has resulted in most of the live births after transplantation, vitrification of ovarian tissue is an emerging focus of investigation, and the first live birth after transplantation of vitrified-warmed tissue was recently reported [34, 35].

To date orthotopic or heterotopic transplantation is the only available option to restore fertility using cryopreserved ovarian tissue, as other techniques require additional research before becoming available for humans.

The transplant is usually performed when the patient is willing to get pregnant, with the permission of the oncologists, as the duration of ovarian tissue transplanted is limited in time [36]. For the same reason, not all the fragments of ovarian cortex available are thawed and transplanted at the same time, when feasible.

Transplantation can take place either into the pelvic cavity, in the orthotopic transplant, or in alternative sites in the heterotopic transplant (Table 4.2). In consideration of the low invasivity, the subcutaneous site is sometimes associated with transplantation at the orthotopic site [37, 38].

There are essentially two techniques of orthotopic (in the pelvis) transplantation that may be used depending on the presence or not of at least one remaining ovary. If at least one ovary is present, the technique starts with decortication of the ovary in order to have access to the medulla and its vascular network. Ovarian cortical pieces are then fixed to or placed on the medulla. If ovaries were previously removed, a peritoneal pocket to place ovarian fragments may be created. Transplantation can be performed at the peritoneal site even if a non-functioning ovary is still in place, in addition to the transplant at the ovarian site or as unique location [39]. Some authors

Table 4.2 Orthotopic versus heterotopic ovarian transplantation

	Heterotopic transplantation	Orthotopic transplantation
Advantages	Easy transplantation procedure Easy access for follicular monitoring and oocyte collection	Possibility of natural conception Restoration of fertility widely demonstrated Favorable environment for follicular development
Disadvantages	Restoration of fertility demonstrated only in one case IVF procedure required Effect of the local environment on oocyte quality unknown	Invasive transplantation procedure

performed transplantation at the ovarian site [40–42], other groups used the perito-neal window [32, 43–46], and lastly there were some associating the two techniques [47–53]. Transplantation can be performed either using laparotomy [40–42, 44], laparoscopy [32, 43, 45–50, 52], or a combination of the two techniques [51], while some authors suggest the possible use of robotic surgery [54].

Even if ovarian tissue is amenable to avascular transplantation the potential of revascularization of the graft is the most important factor for success, because it establishes the survival rate of the follicle pool within the graft. As for the preven-tion of ischemic damage, Donnez proposed the "two-step" approach. During the preparatory laparoscopy (7 days before reimplantation), he created a peritoneal window with the goal of inducing angiogenesis and neo-vascularization in the area, by triggering endogenous processes of new vessel formation. During the second intervention, he reimplanted the frozen–thawed ovarian fragments where a newly formed vascular network in the peritoneal window was clearly seen [47]. Demeestere suggested to associate at the "two-step" technique a subcutaneous heterotopic trans-plantation at the abdominal site; Piver and Roux suggested to add small pieces 1–2 mm of thawed ovarian cortex during the first surgery to facilitate the production of angiogenic factors [48, 50]. As an alternative, Revel proposed the use of micro-organs (MOs), fragments whose thickness are about 300–350 mM, that remain viable and transcribe specific genes for long periods both in culture and when implanted into hosts [44]. Callejo proposed to use angiogenic factors to improve the vascularization of the implant and its quality; he used a gel preparation of PRP (plasma rich in platelets) to impregnate the thawed cubes of ovarian tissue and to fill the peritoneal pockets where the fragments were placed [45].

The risk of reintroducing malignant cells theoretically exists in breast cancer patients [43]. Breast cancer can metastasize to the ovaries, more commonly in advanced-stage cancer, even if the development of an ovarian tumor is more likely to be of primary ovarian origin than a breast cancer metastasis [55]. A special atten-tion should be reserved to BRCA mutation carriers.

Different studies based on the examination of cryopreserved ovarian tissue from women with breast cancer using both conventional histology and immunohisto-chemistry revealed no evidence of malignant cell involvement [56–58].

On the other hand, in a large review of 5,571 female autopsies, Kyono evidenced ovarian metastases in 24.2 % of breast cancer patients [59]. As these data were obtained as results of autopsies, they reflect the risk of ovarian involvement in patients with advanced breast cancer; patients who are offered ovarian tissue cryopreservation have a minimal risk of dissemination and ovarian involvement. Anyway, the results from this study suggest that a great caution is necessary when transplanting the tissue of breast cancer patients. A pilot study by Donnez demonstrated that cryopreserved ovarian tissue from patients with advanced-stage breast cancer may contain cells expressing the MGB2 gene, even if the real malignant potential of these cells is not yet known [60]. Ernst reported a legal termination of pregnancy due to breast cancer recurrence in a patient who spontaneously conceived after ovarian tissue transplant, even though the authors considered unlikely that the transplanted tissue had any effect on the recurrence of cancer [61]. Apart from the possibility of tumor contamination of the cryopreserved tissue, the return of natural ovarian function may have an impact on the course of breast cancer.

For patients with a potential risk of having malignant cells in their cryopreserved ovarian tissue, other options could be the follicle culture with in vitro maturation [33, 62], the grafting of isolated follicles [63], ovarian tissue purging to eliminate malignant cells [64], and artificial ovaries composed of primordial follicles combined with disease-free stromal elements or placed in an alginate matrigel matrix [65].

The analysis of the recovery of ovarian function after ovarian tissue transplantation is difficult because of the lack of reports in the literature which indicate how many patients in the world have been subjected to the procedure. Anyway the regain of endocrine function has been described in all published cases of ovarian transplantation, both orthotopic and heterotopic. Ovarian function has been demonstrated to persist up to 7 years after transplantation with a mean duration of 4–5 years [36].

To date almost 30 live births have been reported worldwide after orthotopic ovarian transplant [39–42, 44–53, 66–68], whereas heterotopic graft has led to one twin pregnancy [69], a biochemical pregnancy [38], and four spontaneous pregnancies with three live births as a result of a reactivation of the native ovary [70]. Most pregnancies were obtained from women younger than 30 years at the time of cryopreservation, as the age at ovarian retrieval is one of the most important predictive factors, since the follicular reserve is age dependent. After orthotopic transplant, more than 50 % of women were able to conceive naturally and this fact constitutes a good point in favor of orthotopic reimplantation. Pregnancy outcomes were similar to those in the general population and all the babies were healthy.

In conclusion, the effectiveness of ovarian tissue cryopreservation and transplantation in terms of endocrine function and fertility restoration has been proven, and even if still experimental, OTC is a good option to preserve fertility in breast cancer patients when ovarian stimulation is not feasible.

4.4 Ovarian Suppression with GnRH Analogs

A GnRH analog (GnRHa) is a molecule derived from the native GnRH by substituting some of the amino acids.

GnRH agonists initially have a flare-up effect – stimulating the release of FSH and LH – while after chronic administration result in a downregulation of GnRH receptors and in a long-term desensitization of the pituitary cells producing gonadotropins. The final effect is decreasing FSH secretion and thus suppressing ovarian function, follicular development, and E2 secretion.

The rationale behind the use of GnRH agonists to reduce the gonadal toxicity of chemotherapy is based on the following issues:

- Chemotherapy mostly affects tissues with a rapid cellular turnover: a state of inhibition during exposure to cytotoxic drugs may protect the ovaries.
- Hypoestrogenism could imply a reduced ovarian perfusion and a lower dose of gonadotoxic agents reaching the ovaries.
- Cyclophosphamide, and chemotherapy in general, alters the physiological quiescent status of the primordial follicles, inducing an increase in follicle activation, growth, and apoptosis. The derived damage to follicular ovarian reserve and the consequent reduction in estrogens, inhibin, and AMH cause an increase in FSH which further increases the accelerated recruitment of primordial follicles. Inhibiting FSH release by GnRH agonists can stop this vicious mechanism, otherwise called "ovarian reservoir burnout" [71]. Ovarian functional suppression through GnRH agonist administration has to be reached before the start of chemotherapy and should last during the entire period of cytotoxic treatment.

The advantages of this "medical" approach are the potential preservation of the overall ovarian function, the drug availability in every cancer care unit, and the fact that this method does not require an invasive procedure. Furthermore, it could be combined with other fertility preservation strategies with an expected improvement of fertility outcome. On the other hand, a complete onco-fertility counseling should explain to the patient the possibility of side effects related to the climacteric symptoms. An "add-back" therapy with estrogens, only through local formulations, could be considered in order to improve the overall quality of life and the therapeutic compliance.

A few data are available on the long-term efficacy of this strategy. The ASCO and the European Society for Medical Oncology (ESMO) guidelines still consider this strategy experimental [1, 72]. The potential protective effect of GnRH agonists for the prevention of chemotherapy-induced premature ovarian failure in breast cancer patients has been investigated in observational and phase II studies that showed an overall 91 % of reversibility. Several studies investigated the efficacy of GnRH agonists to preserve ovarian function in breast cancer patients candidates for chemotherapy; they were performed randomizing the patients to

Table 4.3 Meta-analysis about the use of GnRH analogs during chemotherapy to preserve gonadal function and fertility

Paper	Number of patients	Number of studies included in the meta-analysis	Main results (GnRHa vs. controls)
Beck-Fruchter (2008)	345	12	91 % preserved ovarian function, 19 % had a pregnancy
Clowse (2009)	178	9	OR 0.68 of ovarian function preservation; 22 % pregnancy vs. 14 % in controls
Bedaiwy (2009)	340	6	OR 3.46 resumption of menses (any improvement of pregnancy rates)
Kim (2010)	124	11	OR 10.57 in preserving ovarian function (not significant in RCT studies)
Chen (2011)	157	4	OR 1.9 resumption of menses (any improvement of pregnancy rates)
Wang (2013)	677	7	OR 2.83 resumption of menses
Yang (2013)	528	5	OR 0.40 of POF, similar rate of resumption of menses
Del Mastro (2014)	765	9	OR 0.43 of POF

receive adjuvant and/or neo-adjuvant chemotherapy in combination with GnRH agonists vs. chemotherapy alone [73–80]. These studies reported conflicting results. Too many variables were involved and could bias the results: target population, type of chemotherapeutic medications, timing of therapies, patient's age and prognosis, baseline ovarian reserve, concomitant subfertility conditions at time of diagnosis, duration of follow-up, definition of ovarian failure, etc. Aiming to overcome this study heterogeneity, the results of these studies have recently been reanalyzed in meta-analysis, and despite some controversies (Table 4.3) they showed a benefit of the administration of GnRH agonists in the prevention of chemotherapy-induced ovarian failure [81–88]. This benefit, however, concerned the resumption of menstrual bleeding and hormonal status, reflecting the steroidogenesis of the ovary. As for fertility, on the contrary, the efficacy of GnRH agonists' administration remains unproven. For this reason, the recently published guidelines of ASCO and ESMO do not recommend this treatment for fertility preservation, but only as a strategy for hormonal ovarian function preservation [1, 72]. Hence, the GnRH analog strategy could be proposed once integrated in a wider scenario where the other fertility preservation options have to be offered.

Conclusion

Considering the impact of infertility on long-term quality of life, all young patients affected by BC potentially facing premature ovarian insufficiency should receive accurate information concerning the available options to preserve their fertility.

References

1. Loren AW, Mangu PB, Beck LN, Brennan L, Magdalinski AJ, Partridge AH, et al. Fertility preservation for patients with cancer: American Society of Clinical Oncology Clinical Practice Guideline Update. J Clin Oncol. 2013;31(19):2500–10.
2. Practice Committee of American Society for Reproductive Medicine. Fertility preservation in patients undergoing gonadotoxic therapy or gonadectomy: a committee opinion. Fertil Steril. 2013;100(5):1214–23.
3. Cakmak H, Rosen MP. Ovarian stimulayion in cancer patients. Fertil Steril. 2013;99: 1476–84.
4. Kasum M, Simunic´ V, Oreskovic´ S. Fertility preservation with ovarian stimulation protocols prior to cancer treatment. Gynecol Endocrinol. 2013;30:182–6.
5. Depalo R, Jayakrishan K, Garruti G. GnRH agonist versus GnRH antagonist in in vitro fertilization for embryo transfer (IVF/ET). Reprod Biol Endocrinol. 2012;13:10–26.
6. Anderson RA, Kinniburg D, Baird DT. Preliminary experience of the use of gonadotrophin-releasing hormone antagonist in ovulation induction/in vitro fertilization prior to cancer treatment. Hum Reprod. 1999;14:2665–8.
7. Humaidan P, Bungum L, Bungum M. Reproductive outcome using a GnRH antagonist (cetrorelix) for luteolysis and follicular synchronization in poor responder IVF/ICSI patients treated with a flexible GnRH antagonist protocol. Reprod Biomed Online 2005;11(6):679–84.
8. Cakmak H, Zamah AM, Katz A. Effective method for emergency fertility preservation: random start controlled ovarian hyperstimulation. Fertil Steril. 2012;98:170–8.
9. von Wolff M, Thaler CJ, Frambach T. Ovarian stimulation to cryopreserve fertilez oocytes in cancer patients can be started in the luteal phase. Fertil Steril. 2009;92:1360–5.
10. Reddy J, Oktay K. Ovarian stimulation and fertility preservation with the use of aromatase inhibitors in women with breast cancer. Fertil Steril. 2012;98:1363–9.
11. Rodriguez-Wallberg KA, Oktay K. Fertility preservation in women with breast cancer. Clin Obstet Gynecol. 2010;53:753–62.
12. Early Breast Cancer Trialists' Collaborative Group. Systemic treatment of early breast cancer by hormonal, cytotoxic, or immune therapy. 133 randomised trials involving 31 000 recurrences and 24 000 deaths among 75 000 women. Lancet. 1992;339:71–85.
13. Oktay K, Buyuk E, Davis O. Fertility preservation in breast cancer patients: IVF and embryo cryopreservation after ovarian stimulation with tamoxifen. Hum Reprod. 2003;18:90–5.
14. Oktay K, Buyuk E, Libertella L. Fertility preservation in breast cancer patients: a prospective controlled comparison of ovarian stimulation with tamoxifen and letrozole for embryo cryopreservation. J Clin Oncol. 2005;23:4347–53.
15. Meirow D, Raanani H, Maman E. Tamoxifen co-administration during controlled ovarian hyperstimulation for in vitro fertilization in breast cancer patients increases the safety of fertility preservation treatment. Fertil Steril. 2014;102:488–95.
16. Smith IE, Dowsett M. Aromatase inhibitors in breast cancer. N Engl J Med. 2003;348:2431–42.
17. Cole PA, Robinson CH. Mechanism and inhibition of cytochrome P-450 aromatase. J Med Chem. 1990;33:2933–42.
18. Mitwally MF, Casper RF. Use of aromatase inhibitor for induction of ovulation in patients with an inadequate response to clomiphene citrate. Fertil Steril. 2001;75:305–9.
19. Fisher SA, Reid RL, Van Vugt DA. A randomized double-blind comparison of the effects of clomiphene citrate and the aromatase inhibitor letrozole on ovulatory function in normal women. Fertil Steril. 2002;78:280–5.
20. Reddy J, Turan V, Bedoschi G. Triggering final oocyte maturation with gonadotropin-releasing hormone agonist (GnRHa) versus human chorionic gonadotropin (hCG) in breast cancer patients undergoing fertility preservation: an extended experience. J Assist Reprod Genet. 2014;31:927–32.

21. Azim AA, Costantini-Ferrando M, Oktay K. Safety of fertility preservation by ovarian stimulation with letrozole and gonadotropis in patients with breast cancer: a prospective controlled study. J Clin Oncol. 2008;26:2630–5.
22. Rodriguez-Wallberg KA, Oktay K. Fertility preservation during cancer treatment: clinical guidelines. Cancer Manag Res. 2014;6:105–17.
23. Johnson LN, Dillon KE, Sammel MD. Response to ovarian stimulation in patients facing gonadotoxic therapy. Reprod Biomed Online. 2013;26:337–44.
24. Rodriguez-Wallberg KA, Oktay K. Fertility preservation and pregnancy in women with and without BRCA mutation-positive breast cancer. Oncologist. 2012;17(11):1409–17. doi:10.1634/theoncologist.2012-0236. Epub 2012 Sep 24.
25. Lin WT, Beattie M, Chen LM. Comparison of age at natural menopause in BRCA1/2 mutation carriers with a non-clinic-based sample of women in northern California. Cancer. 2013;119(9):1652–9.
26. Lee S, Oktay K. Does starting dose of FSH with letrozole improve fertility preservation outcomes in women with breast cancer? Fertil Steril. 2012;98:961–4.
27. Baart EB, Martini E, Eijkemans MJ. Milder ovarian stimulation for in vitro fertilization reduces aneuploidy in the human preimplantation embryo: a randomized controlled trial. Hum Reprod. 2007;22:980–8.
28. Lee S, Ozkavukcu S, Heytens E. Value of early referral to fertility preservation in young women with breast cancer. Clin Oncol. 2010;28:4683–6.
29. Newton H, Aubard Y, Rutherford A, Sharma V, Gosden R. Low temperature storage and grafting of human ovarian tissue. Hum Reprod. 1996;11:1487–91.
30. Schmidt KT, Nyboe Andersen A, Greve T, Ernst E, Loft A, Yding Andersen C. Fertility in cancer patients after cryopreservation of one ovary. Reprod Biomed Online. 2013;26:272–9.
31. Meirow D, Fasouliotis SJ, Nugent D, Schenker JG, Gosden RG, Rutherford AJ. A laparoscopic technique for obtaining ovarian cortical biopsy specimens for fertility conservation in patients with cancer. Fertil Steril. 1999;71:948–51.
32. Dittrich R, Lotz L, Keck G, Hoffmann I, Mueller A, Beckmann MW, van der Ven H, Montag M. Live birth after ovarian tissue autotransplantation following overnight transportation before cryopreservation. Fertil Steril. 2012;97(2):387–90.
33. Fasano G, Moffa F, Dechène J, Englert Y, Demeestere I. Vitrification of in vitro matured oocytes collected from antral follicles at the time of ovarian tissue cryopreservation. Reprod Biol Endocrinol. 2011;9:150.
34. Amorim CA, Curaba M, Van Langendonckt A, Dolmans MM, Donnez J. Vitrification as an alternative means of cryopreserving ovarian tissue. Reprod Biomed Online. 2011;23:160–86.
35. Kawamura K, Cheng Y, Suzuki N, et al. Hippo signaling disruption and Akt stimulation of ovarian follicles for infertility treatment. Proc Natl Acad Sci U S A. 2013;110:17474–9.
36. Kim SS. Assessment of long term endocrine function after transplantation of frozen-thawed human ovarian tissue to the heterotopic site: 10 year longitudinal follow-up study. J Assist Reprod Genet. 2012;29(6):489–93.
37. Demeestere I, Simon P, Buxant F, Robin V, Fernandez SA, Centner J, Delbaere A, Englert Y. Ovarian function and spontaneous pregnancy after combined heterotopic and orthotopic cryopreserved ovarian tissue transplantation in a patient previously treated with bone marrow transplantation: case report. Hum Reprod. 2006;21:2010–4.
38. Rosendahl M, Loft A, Byskov AG, Ziebe S, Schmidt KT, Andersen AN, Ottosen C, Andersen CY. Biochemical pregnancy after fertilization of an oocyte aspirated from a heterotopic autotransplant of cryopreserved ovarian tissue: case report. Hum Reprod. 2006;21:2006–9.
39. Donnez J, Dolmans MM, Pellicer A, Diaz-Garcia C, Sanchez Serrano M, Schmidt KT, Ernst E, Luyckx V, Andersen CY. Restoration of ovarian activity and pregnancy after transplantation of cryopreserved ovarian tissue: a review of 60 cases of reimplantation. Fertil Steril. 2013; 99(6):1503–13.
40. Meirow D, Levron J, Eldar-Geva T, Hardan I, Fridman E, Zalel Y, Schiff E, Dor J. Pregnancy after transplantation of cryopreserved ovarian tissue in a patient with ovarian failure after chemotherapy. N Engl J Med. 2005;353:318–21.

41. Sanchez-Serrano M, Crespo J, Mirabet V, Cobo AC, Escriba MJ, Simon C, et al. Twins born after transplantation of human ovarian cortical tissue and oocyte vitrification. Fertil Steril. 2010;93:268.e11–3.
42. Silber SJ. Ovary cryopreservation and transplantation for fertility preservation. Mol Hum Reprod. 2012;18(2):59–67.
43. Oktay K. Ovarian tissue cryopreservation and transplantation: preliminary findings and implications for cancer patients. Hum Reprod Update. 2001;7:526–34.
44. Revel A, Laufer N, Ben Meir A, Lebovich M, Mitrani E. Micro-organ ovarian transplantation enables pregnancy: a case report. Hum Reprod. 2011;26:1097–103.
45. Callejo J, Salvador C, González-Nuñez S, Almeida L, Rodriguez L, Marqués L, Valls A, Lailla JM. Live birth in a woman without ovaries after autograft of frozen-thawed ovarian tissue combined with growth factors. J Ovarian Res. 2013;6(1):33.
46. Donnez J, Jadoul P, Pirard C, Hutchings G, Demylle D, Squifflet J, Smitz J, Dolmans MM. Live birth after transplantation of frozen-thawed ovarian tissue after bilateral oophorectomy for benign disease. Fertil Steril. 2012;98(3):720–5.
47. Donnez J, Dolmans MM, Demylle D, Jadoul P, Pirard C, Squifflet J, Martinez-Madrid B, van Langendonckt A. Livebirth after orthotopic transplantation of cryopreserved ovarian tissue. Lancet. 2004;364(9443):1405–10.
48. Demeestere I, Simon P, Emiliani S, Delbaere A, Englert Y. Fertility preservation: successful transplantation of cryopreserved ovarian tissue in a young patient previously treated for Hodgkin's disease. Oncologist. 2007;12(12):1437–42.
49. Piver P, Amiot C, Agnani G, Pech J, Rohrlich PS, Vidal E. et al. Two pregnancies obtained after a new technique of autotransplantation of cryopreserved ovarian tissue. In: 25th annual meeting of ESHRE, 28 June–1 July, 2009. Amsterdam: Oxford University Press. Hum Reprod; 2009.
50. Roux C, Amiot C, Agnani G, Aubard Y, Rohrlich PS, Piver P. Live birth after ovarian tissue autograft in a patient with sickle cell disease treated by allogeneic bone marrow transplantation. Fertil Steril. 2010;93:2413.
51. Andersen CY, Rosendahl M, Byskov AG, Loft A, Ottosen C, Dueholm M, Schmidt KL, Andersen AN, Ernst E. Two successful pregnancies following autotransplantation of frozen/thawed ovarian tissue. Hum Reprod. 2008;23:2266–72.
52. Revelli A, Marchino G, Dolfin E, Molinari E, Delle Piane L, Salvagno F, Benedetto C. Live birth after orthotopic grafting of autologous cryopreserved ovarian tissue and spontaneous conception in Italy. Fertil Steril. 2013;99(1):227–30.
53. Ernst E, Bergholdt S, Jørgensen JS, Andersen CY. The first woman to give birth to two children following transplantation of frozen/thawed ovarian tissue. Hum Reprod. 2010;25(5):1280–1.
54. Akar ME, Carrello AJ, Jennell JL, Yalcinkaya TM. Robotic-assisted laparoscopic ovarian tissue transplantation. Fertil Steril. 2011;95(3):1120.e5–e8.
55. Bigorie V, Morice P, Duvillard P, Antoine M, Cortez A, Flejou JF, et al. Ovarian metastases from breast cancer: report of 29 cases. Cancer. 2010;116:799–804.
56. Azem F, Hasson J, Ben-Yosef D, Kossoy N, Cohen T, Almog B, Amit A, Lessing JB, Lifschitz-Mercer B. Histologic evaluation of fresh human ovarian tissue before cryopreservation. Int J Gynecol Pathol. 2010;29:19–23.
57. Sanchez-Serrano M, Novella-Maestre E, Rosello-Sastre E, Camarasa N, Teruel J, Pellicer A. Malignant cells are not found in ovarian cortex from breast cancer patients undergoing ovarian cortex cryopreservation. Hum Reprod. 2009;24:2238–43.
58. Rosendahl M, Timmermans Wielenga V, Nedergaard L, Kristensen SG, Ernst E, Rasmussen PE, Anderson M, Schmidt KT, Andersen CY. Cryopreservation of ovarian tissue for fertility preservation: no evidence of malignant cell contamination in ovarian tissue from patients with breast cancer. Fertil Steril. 2011;95:2158–61.
59. Kyono K, Doshida M, Toya M, Sato Y, Akahira J, Sasano H. Potential indications for ovarian autotransplantation based on the analysis of 5,571 autopsy findings of females under the age of 40 in Japan. Fertil Steril. 2010;93:2429–30.
60. Luyckx V, Durant JF, Camboni A, Gilliaux S, Amorim CA, Van Langendonckt A, Irenge LM, Gala JL, Donnez J, Dolmans MM. Is transplantation of cryopreserved ovarian tissue from

patients with advanced-stage breast cancer safe? A pilot study. J Assist Reprod Genet. 2013;30(10):1289–99.
61. Ernst EH, Offersen BV, Andersen CY, Ernst E. Legal termination of a pregnancy resulting from transplanted cryopreserved ovarian tissue due to cancer recurrence. J Assist Reprod Genet. 2013;30(7):975–8.
62. Prasath EB, Chan MLH, Wong WHW, et al. First pregnancy and live birth resulting from cryopreserved embryos obtained from in vitro matured oocytes after oophorectomy in an ovarian cancer patient. Hum Reprod. 2014;29:276–8.
63. Dolmans MM, Martinez-Madrid B, Gadisseux E, Guiot Y, Yuan WY, Torre A, Camboni A, Van Langendonckt A, Donnez J. Short-term transplantation of isolated human ovarian follicles and cortical tissue into nude mice. Reproduction. 2007;134(2):253–62.
64. Schröder CP, Timmer-Bosscha H, Wijchman JG, et al. An in vitro model for purging of tumour cells from ovarian tissue. Hum Reprod. 2004;19:1069–75.
65. Vanacker J, Luyckx V, Dolmans MM, Des Rieux A, Jaeger J, Van Langendonckt A, Donnez J, Amorim CA. Transplantation of an alginate-matrigel matrix containing isolated ovarian cells: first step in developing a biodegradable scaffold to transplant isolated preantral follicles and ovarian cells. Biomaterials. 2012;33(26):6079–85.
66. Demeestere I, Simon P, Moffa F, Delbaere A, Englert Y. Birth of a second healthy girl more than 3 years after cryopreserved ovarian graft. Hum Reprod. 2010;25(6):1590–1. doi:10.1093/humrep/deq096. Epub 2010 Apr 14.
67. Burmeister L, Kovacs GT, Osianlis T. First Australian pregnancy after ovarian tissue cryopreservation and subsequent autotransplantation. Med J Aust. 2013;198(3):158–9.
68. Macklon KT, Jensen AK, Loft A, Ernst E. Andersen CY Treatment history and outcome of 24 deliveries worldwide after autotransplantation of cryopreserved ovarian tissue, including two new Danish deliveries years after autotransplantation. J Assist Reprod Genet. 2014;12.
69. Stern CJ, Toledo MG, Hale LG, Gook DA, Edgar DH. The first Australian experience of heterotopic grafting of cryopreserved ovarian tissue: evidence of establishment of normal ovarian function. Aust N Z J Obstet Gynaecol. 2011;51(3):268–75.
70. Oktay K, Türkçüoğlu I, Rodriguez-Wallberg KA. Four spontaneous pregnancies and three live births following subcutaneous transplantation of frozen banked ovarian tissue: what is the explanation? Fertil Steril. 2011;95(2):804.e7–10.
71. Kalich-Philosoph L, Roness H, Carmely A, Fishel-Bartal M, Ligumsky H, Paglin S, et al. Cyclophosphamide triggers follicle activation and "burnout"; AS101 prevents follicle loss and preserves fertility. Sci Transl Med. 2013;5(185):185ra62.
72. Peccatori FA, Azim Jr HA, Orecchia R, Hoekstra HJ, Pavlidis N, Kesic V, et al. Cancer, pregnancy and fertility: ESMO clinical practice guidelines for diagnosis, treatment and follow-up. Ann Oncol. 2013;24 Suppl 6:vi160–70.
73. Badawy A, Elnashar A, El-Ashry M, Shahat M. Gonadotropin-releasing hormone agonists for prevention of chemotherapy-induced ovarian damage: prospective randomized study. Fertil Steril. 2009;91(3):694–7.
74. Del Mastro L, Boni L, Michelotti A, Gamucci T, Olmeo N, Gori S, et al. Effect of the gonadotropin-releasing hormone analogue triptorelin on the occurrence of chemotherapy-induced early menopause in premenopausal women with breast cancer: a randomized trial. JAMA. 2011;306(3):269–76.
75. Gerber B, von Minckwitz G, Stehle H, Reimer T, Felberbaum R, Maass N, et al. Effect of luteinizing hormone-releasing hormone agonist on ovarian function after modern adjuvant breast cancer chemotherapy: the GBG 37 ZORO study. J Clin Oncol. 2011;29(17):2334–41.
76. Munster PN, Moore AP, Ismail-Khan R, Cox CE, Lacevic M, Gross-King M, et al. Randomized trial using gonadotropin-releasing hormone agonist triptorelin for the preservation of ovarian function during (neo)adjuvant chemotherapy for breast cancer. J Clin Oncol. 2012;30(5):533–8.
77. Sverrisdottir A, Nystedt M, Johansson H, Fornander T. Adjuvant goserelin and ovarian preservation in chemotherapy treated patients with early breast cancer: results from a randomized trial. Breast Cancer Res Treat. 2009;117(3):561–7.

78. Elgindy EA, El-Haieg DO, Khorshid OM, Ismail EI, Abdelgawad M, Sallam HN, et al. Gonadatrophin suppression to prevent chemotherapy induced ovarian damage: a randomized controlled trial. Obstet Gynecol. 2013;121(1):78–86.
79. Halle C, Moore F, et al. Prevention of early menopause study [POEMS] –SWOG S0230. http:// abstracts.asco.org/144/AbstView_144_129172.html. J Clin Oncol 32:5s, 2014 suppl; abstr LBA505.
80. Karimi-Zarchi M, Forat-Yazdi M, Vafaeenasab MR, Nakhaie-Moghadam M, Miratashi-Yazdi A, Teimoori S, Dehghani-Tafti A. Evaluation of the effect of GnRH agonist on menstrual reverse in breast cancer cases treated with cyclophosphamide. Eur Gynaecol Oncol. 2014;35(1):59–61.
81. Kim SS, Lee JR, Jee BC, Suh CS, Kim SH, Ting A, et al. Use of hormonal protection for chemotherapy-induced gonadotoxicity. Clin Obstet Gynecol. 2010;53(4):740–52.
82. Bedaiwy MA, Abou-Setta AM, Desai N, Hurd W, Starks D, El-Nashar SA, et al. Gonadotropin-releasing hormone analog cotreatment for preservation of ovarian function during gonadotoxic chemotherapy: a systematic review and meta-analysis. Fertil Steril. 2011;95(3):906-914. e1-e4.
83. Chen H, Li J, Cui T, Hu L. Adjuvant gonadotropin-releasing hormone analogues for the prevention of chemotherapy induced premature ovarian failure in premenopausal women. Cochrane Database Syst Rev. 2011;(11): CD008018.
84. Wang C, Chen M, Fu F, Huang M. Gonadotropin-releasing hormone analog cotreatment for the preservation of ovarian function during gonadotoxic chemotherapy for breast cancer: a meta-analysis. PLoS One. 2013;8(6):e66360.
85. Yang B, Shi W, Yang J, Liu H, Zhao H, Li X, et al. Concurrent treatment with gonadotropin-releasing hormone agonists for chemotherapy-induced ovarian damage in premenopausal women with breast cancer: a meta-analysis of randomized controlled trials. Breast Edinb Scotl. 2013;22(2):150–7.
86. Clowse ME, Behera MA, Anders CK, Copland S, Coffman CJ. Ovarian preservation by GnRH agonists during chemotherapy: a meta-analysis. J Womens Health (Larchmt). 2009;18:311–9.
87. Del Mastro L, Ceppi M, Poggio F, Bighin C, Peccatori F, Demeestere I, et al. Gonadotropin-releasing hormone analogues for the prevention of chemotherapy-induced premature ovarian failure in cancer women: systematic review and meta-analysis of randomized trials. Cancer Treat Rev. 2014;40(5):675–83.
88. Beck-Fruchter R, Weiss A, Shalev E. GnRH agonist therapy as ovarian protectants in female patients undergoing chemotherapy: a review of the clinical data. Hum Reprod Update. 2008;14(6):553–61.

Giovanni Codacci-Pisanelli, Giovanna Scarfone,
Lino Del Pup, Eleonora Zaccarelli, and Fedro A. Peccatori

5.1   Introduction

The occurrence of cancer in a pregnant woman is one of the most distressing medical experiences [2]. The woman, the attending gynaecologist and the medical oncologist are faced with a frightening diagnosis which is made even worse since it involves two subjects: the mother and the baby. In some situations there may be a conflict between the two [24, 25], but in most cases such a conflict is only apparent [31] and the mother

G. Codacci-Pisanelli, MD, PhD
Fertility and Procreation Unit, European Institute of Oncology,
Via Ripamonti, 435, Milan 20141, Italy

Department of Medicine, Surgery and Biotechnology, University of Rome
"la Sapienza", Corso della Repubblica, 79, Latina 04100, Italy
e-mail: giovanni.codaccipisanelli@ieo.it

G. Scarfone, MD
Department of Obstetrics and Gynecology, IRCCS Ospedale Maggiore
Policlinico, Via Commenda, 8, Milan 20145, Italy
e-mail: giotop@katamail.com

L. Del Pup, MD
Department of Gynecologic Oncology, National Institute of Cancer,
Via Franco Gallini, 2, Aviano (PN) 33081, Italy
e-mail: delpuplino@libero.it

E. Zaccarelli, MD
Department of Medicine, Surgery and Biotechnology, University of Rome
"la Sapienza", Corso della Repubblica, 79, Latina 04100, Italy
e-mail: ele.zaccarelli@gmail.com

F.A. Peccatori, MD, PhD (✉)
Fertility and Procreation Unit, European Institute of Oncology,
Via Ripamonti, 435, Milan 20141, Italy
e-mail: fedro.peccatori@ieo.it

© Springer International Publishing Switzerland 2015
N. Biglia, F.A. Peccatori (eds.), *Breast Cancer, Fertility Preservation
and Reproduction*, DOI 10.1007/978-3-319-17278-1_5

can be treated in the most effective way with no disadvantage to the baby [3, 4]. Various malignancies can appear in pregnancy [6, 7, 11, 13, 24, 25, 29, 31]: we will focus on breast cancer.

Several articles have been published that give an authoritative opinion on this subject [1, 2, 6, 7, 21, 22, 28], and the reader is referred to such papers for a detailed description of specific items.

The aim of this chapter is to describe a reasonable approach to treat breast cancer in the different phases of pregnancy: good results can only be obtained through the collaboration of all involved specialists [3, 4], and in this situation it becomes particularly evident that doctors must care for the mother and for the baby, not only treat the tumour [28].

The need to choose the essential diagnostic exams and to limit unnecessary treatments provides an excellent opportunity to evaluate the real use of many procedures that are routinely used in non-pregnant breast cancer patients with no really sound rationale. The same applies to the choice of anticancer agents: in several cases the advantage given by a new drug may be clinically negligible and still cause major toxicity. It is therefore advisable to choose wisely in order to use only agents that will be of real use to both the mother and the foetus.

5.2   Incidence

Cancer during pregnancy is still an unusual event, but unfortunately it is becoming more common and doctors must be prepared to face such a diagnosis.

Childbearing in western world is often postponed by women who choose to fulfil their personal and professional objectives before seeking a pregnancy and accepting the responsibilities it implies.

Age at first delivery therefore overlaps the age at which breast cancer incidence starts to rise sharply, and the two situations may occur simultaneously.

5.3   Diagnosis

Data collected from oncological centres that have a large experience in the treatment of breast cancer in pregnancy show that diagnostic delay is almost inevitable. Doctors must consider the possibility of cancer when visiting pregnant women with uncommon breast findings. The physiological and anatomical modifications occurring in the breast during pregnancy may simulate, or mask, a malignant nodule. In both cases, the identification is more difficult.

5.3.1   Clinical Symptoms

The most common symptom of a malignant breast tumour in pre-menopausal women is the appearance of a non-painful lump: more rarely the first sign is a palpable axillary node. It is of course difficult to distinguish a benign nodule (typically a fibroadenoma) from cancer based on physical examination, and clinicians must always keep in mind the possibility of a non-benign lesion.

5.3.2 Reasons for Diagnostic Delay

A growing nodule in the breast is difficult to interpret in a pregnant woman, when the whole body and the breasts in particular undergo relevant changes in size and in consistency. The low incidence of breast cancer in young women and, in a certain sense, the more or less unconscious refusal of diagnosing a malignant tumour in a pregnant woman will often result in a missed or delayed diagnosis.

5.3.3 Radiology

Ionising radiations are among the best known mutagenic and teratogenic agents: their use during pregnancy should be limited to a minimum, or rather avoided whenever possible. Mammography using a radiological shelter to protect the uterus is feasible and safe for the foetus: this technique has the highest sensitivity to detect microcalcifications. Its use in pre-menopausal women is however less effective than in older patients. In pregnant women this exam can generally be postponed and performed after delivery. Contrast agents also raise some concerns about safety for the foetus. We therefore totally agree that in pregnant women "imaging should be used … only when the benefits outweigh the risks" [38].

5.3.4 Ultrasound

Even if ultrasound scans do not have any role in screening, they provide a detailed evaluation of size and of other characteristics of breast nodules. Furthermore, Doppler techniques add reliable indications on blood flow making a differential diagnosis between benign and malignant lesions easier.

5.3.5 Magnetic Resonance

This technique does not involve the use of ionising radiations and is therefore not contraindicated, but the information it provides is generally not essential for treatment and this exam may be avoided in pregnant women with breast cancer. The main issue remains the false-positive rate during pregnancy and the potential foetal toxicity of gadolinium.

5.3.6 Biopsy

A tumour sample suitable for histological examination can be easily obtained by a core needle biopsy. In most cases the amount of tissue is sufficient to perform not only basic histological analysis, but also to obtain information about the biological features of the tumour, such as hormone receptor status, HER2 overexpression or amplification and proliferation rate.

Local anaesthesia implies no danger to the mother nor to the baby, and even general anaesthesia (which is generally not required for diagnostic purposes) can be safely performed during pregnancy.

Fine needle aspiration, due to cellular changes in the breast caused by hormones, may be difficult to interpret and is therefore not recommended [2].

5.4   Prognosis

Breast cancer that occurs during pregnancy is not intrinsically and biologically different from the same disease occurring in non-pregnant women. A recent paper compared the biological characteristics (grading, hormone receptors, proliferative index and HER2 overexpression) and did not find any relevant difference between cancers occurring in pregnancy when compared with breast cancer in a comparable population of young women. The histological and biological modifications that occur in the breast, however, might justify the worse prognosis of breast cancer presenting during pregnancy or shortly after delivery [8, 35].

The main difficulty in management and the worse results that are often reported possibly derive from the diagnostic delay which is mostly due to the reasons described above.

5.5   Treatment Options

The choice of the appropriate treatment requires sound oncological and obstetrical competence: abortion may appear as the most sensible choice in order to give the mother the best opportunities. Even if this may be tolerable when cancer is diagnosed in the first trimester of pregnancy, termination may not be necessary in later phases. Let us stress how clinical expertise may solve any moral issue.

The risk associated with anticancer treatment depends on the phase in which cancer is diagnosed. Surgery can be safely performed even in the first weeks. Syst emic medical treatment with anticancer drugs is certainly more dangerous, but it should be considered that the placenta protects the baby and effectively prevents foetal exposure to circulating anticancer agents. Placenta, however, does not give any protection from ionising radiations.

5.5.1   Surgery

The most reliable evidence on the safety of surgery (and of general anaesthesia) in pregnancy derives from the large number of procedures that have been performed in pregnant women for emergencies. Breast surgery, if clinically indicated, is therefore feasible. The reason why surgical removal of breast cancer is generally not performed during pregnancy is linked to the treatment strategy that is preferentially based on a pre-operative (neoadjuvant) chemotherapy. Surgery is therefore often delayed and performed after delivery. Not only is breast surgery feasible during pregnancy: it must be stressed that any type of procedure is possible. There is no reason to consider mastectomy as the procedure of choice: partial breast removal, if indicated, can be safely performed in a pregnant woman. Radiotherapy to the breast (and to adjacent tissues if indicated) can then be safely delayed and administered after delivery (see below).

Sentinel lymph node analyses performed in non-pregnant women showed that the dose of radiation that the foetus would receive as a consequence of radioactive identification of an axillary lymph node is very low [15, 16, 34], so there is no reason to withhold this procedure in pregnant women if clinically indicated.

5.5.2 Radiotherapy

Radiotherapy has evident mutagenic and teratogenic effects that are particularly dangerous in the first trimester [19]. Concerning breast cancer treatment, in principle it is possible to administer radiotherapy to the breast and effectively shield the uterus and therefore the baby, but this is not performed in clinical practice. What we actually see is that pregnant women receive adjuvant chemotherapy after surgery for 12–16 weeks. Similarly to what is implemented in non-pregnant women, adjuvant radiation is preferentially administered after the end of chemotherapy and therefore after delivery.

5.5.3 Chemotherapy

Most traditional anticancer agents act by inhibiting the proliferation of malignant cells, but they cannot distinguish between normal and cancer cells. Foetal growth is mostly due to processes of cell proliferation that are identical to those used by cancer cells. Foetal tissues are therefore especially sensitive to antiproliferative treatment [20]. Even agents that have no antiproliferative activity may cause serious damages to the developing baby. Thus, it is easy to understand that for a long time doctors refused to administer chemotherapy, or specific anticancer agents [21], to pregnant women.

Nonetheless, this principle has been challenged in recent years [22].

Today there are enough clinical evidences, supported by pre-clinical data, that confirm the protective role of the placenta in reducing foetal exposure to toxic agents. This organ is able to filter maternal blood and to actively block the passage of chemotherapy drugs, particularly those which are substrates for ABC transporters. These observations were then combined with pharmacological data that suggested that the best way to exploit the protective role of the placenta would be to avoid high peak plasma concentrations also considering the altered pharmacokinetics of anthracyclines in pregnant women [33, 36, 37]. This is the rationale behind the choice of weekly drug administration: the lower dose administered in comparison with a protocol involving a 21-day cycle is definitely less toxic to the baby while the antitumour activity is equivalent [27]. Combination chemotherapy, which is the standard for non-pregnant women, can also be used during pregnancy [18] even if monotherapy is generally preferred. Anthracyclines [3, 4, 23, 33] and taxanes [12, 39, 40] are among the most widely used traditional anticancer agents.

It is important to note that when talking about "chemotherapy" we must also include drugs administered to reduce the unpleasant side effects of treatment, particularly vomiting. Serotonin receptor antagonists, particularly ondansetron, may be safely used during pregnancy [26], while steroid administration should be limited and methylprednisolone rather than dexametasone should be used for its lower transplacental transfer.

5.5.4   Hormonal Treatment

The idea of chemotherapy during pregnancy raises an obvious concern, but it is important to consider that hormones may be as dangerous to the foetus. No hormonal agent (tamoxifen [10] or oestrogen receptor modulators, aromatase inhibitors, inhibitors of LH release) can be used during pregnancy. They should not be used during lactation either.

5.5.5   Biological Agents (Trastuzumab, Lapatinib)

These are the anticancer agents most recently introduced in clinical practice and they are often considered less toxic than traditional anticancer agents. Trastuzumab is the only "biological" agent that has been extensively used for adjuvant treatment of breast cancer during pregnancy, but unfortunately and rather unexpectedly it proved too toxic for use in this setting since it causes oligo- or anhydramnios [5–7, 39, 40]. At the moment safety concerns, also based on pre-clinical data [30], suggest that systemic biological agents should not be used during pregnancy as even intravitreal injections raised concerns [17].

5.5.6   Metastatic Disease

Treatment of metastatic disease is included in this paragraph since almost by definition it can only be treated by systemic therapy. Radiotherapy can be used for palliation of specific symptoms due to bone involvement or to brain metastases. Readers are referred to other publications that give more details on the treatment of metastatic breast cancer during pregnancy [3, 4]. We will focus on specific problems encountered in this condition.

While localised breast cancer implies a relatively good prognosis and treatment is relatively standardised, the approach to metastatic disease is more heterogeneous. Treatment must be tailored on the basis of prognosis, of the potential damage to the foetus and of the real benefit that can be offered in terms of survival and of symptoms palliation. Some specific problems do exist and imply, for example, the need to maintain an adequate liver function in order to allow foetal growth. It is not our aim to discuss rare and dreadful situations that can occur, but again we want to give an indication on reasonable approaches to pregnancy complicated by metastatic breast cancer.

The patient must be informed about the prognosis, the real objective of chemotherapy and by the possible foetal toxicity. In specific situations, when cancer is diagnosed relatively early during gestation, it may be reasonable to delay chemotherapy in a metastatic but asymptomatic patient.

Therapy does not substantially differ from what has been suggested for localised cancer: weekly anthracyclines or paclitaxel are effective and safe treatments that show excellent antitumour activity.

5.6   Attitudes

As already mentioned, cancer treatment in pregnancy requires a careful balance between the necessities of the mother and the protection of the foetus. As these undergo relevant variations during the different stages of pregnancy, the best treatment varies during the course of treatment.

5.6.1   First Trimester

This is the most delicate phase of foetal development and at the same time postponing treatment until after delivery is hardly acceptable. On the other hand, chemotherapy and radiotherapy administered in this phase are associated with the highest risk of serious foetal malformations. For this reason, pregnancy interruption is generally suggested as the most sensible approach. In motivated and well-informed patients with metastatic disease, as already mentioned, it may be possible to delay treatment for some weeks waiting for a phase of foetal development that does not contraindicate chemotherapy.

5.6.2   Second and Third Trimester

During this phase organogenesis is mostly completed and tissues are less sensitive to the antiproliferative effect of drugs. At the same time the placenta is more effective as a filter and protects the foetus. It is therefore possible to administer chemotherapy, starting from the 16th week of pregnancy, up to 35th. After this time it is generally possible to induce delivery as the baby is now sufficiently mature.

Even if a gestational age of 32 weeks is usually sufficient for a good neonatal outcome in terms of survival, subtle anomalies in neurodevelopment have been described even for late premature babies, that is, babies born between 34 and 36 weeks. Thus, a wise balance between anticipated delivery and maternal wellbeing should be pursued.

5.7   Foetal Outcomes

A reason of concern about administering chemotherapy during pregnancy is the possibility of long-term effects on physical and psychological development. This is particularly worrying since acute toxicities are relatively easy to identify, while long-term toxicities require a careful and prolonged follow-up. This painstaking work has however been carried out and all the evidence suggests that children exposed to chemotherapy in utero do not show any developmental impairment.

At present, the most important aspect is to avoid what was properly defined as "iatrogenic prematurity" [36, 37]. Careful obstetrical monitoring should be carried out in order to prolong pregnancy. Early delivery, rather than chemotherapy, seems to be the principal cause of altered development observed in some studies.

5.8   Breastfeeding

Most agents administered to lactating women can be excreted in milk, and chemotherapy or hormonal agents are no exception. Some anticancer drugs can be administered in reduced doses at weekly intervals (a schedule often used for anthracyclines and for taxanes) or as a continuous infusion (which actually only applies to fluorouracil) and plasma concentrations and therefore milk concentrations are very low [9, 14]. The drugs ingested by the baby through breastfeeding undergo liver passage and presumably extensive degradation. No data are however available concerning the ability of the immature liver to effectively degrade ingested molecules even if some reassuring data are available for thiopurine [14]. It is therefore advisable that women undergoing chemotherapy do not breastfeed their children [32].

It must be stressed, however, that this veto is only limited to the time during which medical treatment is administered. This does not extend to successive pregnancies and it may be worth underlining here that a previous chemotherapy, and even radiation therapy to the breast, is by no means a reason to prevent lactation at a later time.

The possibility of pregnancy after cancer is extensively discussed in a different chapter and will not be further analysed here.

Conclusions

The occurrence of cancer during pregnancy remains a challenging experience for the woman and for the attending physicians. Making a decision sometimes implies choosing between the interest of the mother and that of the foetus, but this situation is actually much less frequent than generally imagined. All doctors involved in caring for a pregnant woman with cancer (obstetricians, oncologist, paediatrician) must be fully aware of all the therapeutic possibilities available. This is a fundamental requirement to avoid unnecessary damage to the foetus and offer the best treatment to the mother.

References

1. Amant F, et al. Breast cancer in pregnancy: recommendations of an international consensus meeting. Eur J Cancer. 2010;46(18):3158–68.
2. Amant F, et al. Breast cancer in pregnancy. Lancet. 2012;379(9815):570–9.
3. Azim HA, et al. Anthracyclines for gestational breast cancer: course and outcome of pregnancy. Ann Oncol. 2008;19(8):1511–2.
4. Azim HA, et al. Treatment of metastatic breast cancer during pregnancy: we need to talk! Breast. 2008;17(4):426–8.
5. Azim HA, et al. Breast cancer and pregnancy: how safe is trastuzumab? Nat Rev Clin Oncol. 2009;6(6):367–70.
6. Azim HA, et al. Treatment of cancer during pregnancy with monoclonal antibodies: a real challenge. Exp Rev Clin Immun. 2010;6(6):821–6.
7. Azim HA, et al. Treatment of the pregnant mother with cancer: a systematic review on the use of cytotoxic, endocrine, targeted agents and immunotherapy during pregnancy. Part II: hematological tumors. Cancer Treat Rev. 2010;36(2):110–21.
8. Azim HA, et al. Prognosis of pregnancy-associated breast cancer: a meta-analysis of 30 studies. Cancer Treat Rev. 2012;38(7):834–42.
9. Begg EJ, et al. Studying drugs in human milk: time to unify the approach. J Hum Lact. 2002;18(4):323–32.
10. Braems G, et al. Use of tamoxifen before and during pregnancy. Oncologist. 2011;16(11):1547–51.
11. Brenner B, et al. Haematological cancers in pregnancy. Lancet. 2012;379(9815):580–7.
12. Cardonick E, et al. Maternal and fetal outcomes of taxane chemotherapy in breast and ovarian cancer during pregnancy: case series and review of the literature. Ann Oncol. 2012;23(12):3016–23.
13. Daryanani D, et al. Pregnancy and early-stage melanoma. Cancer. 2003;97(9):2248–53.
14. Gardiner SJ, et al. Exposure to thiopurine drugs through breast milk is low based on metabolite concentrations in mother-infant pairs. Br J Clin Pharmacol. 2006;62(4):453–6.
15. Gentilini O, et al. Safety of sentinel node biopsy in pregnant patients with breast cancer. Ann Oncol. 2004;15(9):1348–51.
16. Gentilini O, et al. Sentinel lymph node biopsy in pregnant patients with breast cancer. Eur J Nucl Med Mol Imaging. 2010;37(1):78–83.
17. Georgalas I, et al. Safety of intravitreal anti-VEGFs during pregnancy is unclear. BMJ. 2012;345:e4526.
18. Hahn KME, et al. Treatment of pregnant breast cancer patients and outcomes of children exposed to chemotherapy in utero. Cancer. 2006;107(6):1219–26.
19. Kal HB, et al. Radiotherapy during pregnancy: fact and fiction. Lancet Oncol. 2005;6(5):328–33.
20. Leslie KK, et al. Chemotherapeutic drugs in pregnancy. Obstet Gynecol Clin North Am. 2005;32(4):627–40.
21. Loibl S, et al. Breast carcinoma during pregnancy. International recommendations from an expert meeting. Cancer. 2006;106(2):237–46.
22. Loibl S, et al. Treatment of breast cancer during pregnancy: an observational study. Lancet Oncol. 2012;13(9):887–96.
23. Mir O, et al. Chemotherapy for breast cancer during pregnancy: is epirubicin safe? Ann Oncol. 2008;19(10):1814–5.
24. Morice P, et al. Gynaecological cancers in pregnancy. Lancet. 2012;379(9815):558–69.
25. Morice P, et al. Cancer in pregnancy: a challenging conflict of interest. Lancet. 2012;379(9815):495–6.
26. Pasternak B, et al. Ondansetron in pregnancy and risk of adverse fetal outcomes. N Engl J Med. 2013;368(9):814–23.
27. Peccatori FA, et al. Weekly epirubicin in the treatment of gestational breast cancer (GBC). Breast Cancer Res Treat. 2009;115(3):591–4.

28. Peccatori FA, et al. Cancer, pregnancy and fertility: ESMO Clinical Practice Guidelines for diagnosis, treatment and follow-up. Ann Oncol. 2013;24 Suppl 6:vi160–70.
29. Pentheroudakis G, et al. Cancer and pregnancy: poena magna, not anymore. Eur J Cancer. 2006;42(2):126–40.
30. Pentsuk N, et al. An interspecies comparison of placental antibody transfer: new insights into developmental toxicity testing of monoclonal antibodies. Birth Defects Res B Dev Reprod Toxicol. 2009;86(4):328–44.
31. Pereg D, et al. Cancer in pregnancy: gaps, challenges and solutions. Cancer Treat Rev. 2008;34(4):302–12.
32. Pistilli B, et al. Chemotherapy, targeted agents, antiemetics and growth-factors in human milk: how should we counsel cancer patients about breastfeeding? Cancer Treat Rev. 2013;39(3): 207–11.
33. Ryu RJ, et al. Pharmacokinetics of doxorubicin in pregnant women. Cancer Chemother Pharmacol. 2014;73(4):789–97.
34. Spanheimer PM, et al. Measurement of uterine radiation exposure from lymphoscintigraphy indicates safety of sentinel lymph node biopsy during pregnancy. Ann Surg Oncol. 2009; 16(5):1143–7.
35. Stensheim H, et al. Cause-specific survival for women diagnosed with cancer during pregnancy or lactation: a registry-based cohort study. J Clin Oncol. 2009;27(1):45–51.
36. Van Calsteren K, et al. Cancer during pregnancy: an analysis of 215 patients emphasizing the obstetrical and the neonatal outcomes. J Clin Oncol. 2010;28(4):683–9.
37. Van Calsteren K, et al. Pharmacokinetics of chemotherapeutic agents in pregnancy: a preclinical and clinical study. Acta Obstet Gynecol Scand. 2010;89(10):1338–45.
38. Wang PI, et al. Imaging of pregnant and lactating patients: part 1, evidence-based review and recommendations. AJR Am J Roentgenol. 2012;198(4):778–84.
39. Zagouri F, et al. Taxanes for breast cancer during pregnancy: a systematic review. Clin Breast Cancer. 2013;13(1):16–23.
40. Zagouri F, et al. Trastuzumab administration during pregnancy: a systematic review and meta-analysis. Breast Cancer Res Treat. 2013;137(2):349–57.

Pregnancy After Breast Cancer

6

Nicoletta Biglia, Nicoletta Tomasi Cont,
Valentina Bounous, Marta d'Alonzo, and Silvia Pecchio

6.1   Introduction

Receiving cancer diagnosis can be devastating for many patients but thanks to advances in cancer therapies it is not a death sentence anymore. Cancer survival rates are increasing and life after cancer is a real chance for many patients worldwide. In Europe, about one third of cancer patients have a relative 5-year survival rate greater than 80 % [1]. Similar survival rates are seen in the United States, Canada and Australia. Lower survival rates in developing countries are most likely due to late diagnosis and limited availability of up-to-date standard treatments [2, 3].

In Italy, every day about 30 new cases of cancer are diagnosed in patients below the age of 40 years and many of them are women with breast cancer. About 10 % of breast cancer diagnosis occurs in patients younger than 40 years [4].

Breast cancer in young women is frequently more aggressive than tumours diagnosed in older women. Often metastases at loco-regional lymph nodes are detected at diagnosis and biological and molecular characteristics identify phenotypes at poor prognosis [5]. As a consequence, systemic treatments in addition to local therapy are frequently recommended. In spite of this, poorer survival rates and higher risk of recurrence are reported in these subgroup of patients [6].

Thanks to adjuvant therapies, overall and disease-free survival are improving over time and most of the patients long survive to breast cancer. Chemotherapy and endocrine therapy extend time to recurrence but, on the other hand, bring about many short- and long-term side effects. Among them, ovarian failure with premature menopause is particularly relevant to young women. In the last few years,

N. Biglia, MD, PhD (✉) • N.T. Cont • V. Bounous • M. d'Alonzo • S. Pecchio
Department of Gynaecology and Obstetrics, University of Torino School
of Medicine, Torino, Italy
e-mail: nicoletta.biglia@unito.it; nicolettatomasi@tiscali.it;
valentinabounous@hotmail.com; martadalonzo@libero.it; silvia86@alice.it

© Springer International Publishing Switzerland 2015
N. Biglia, F.A. Peccatori (eds.), *Breast Cancer, Fertility Preservation
and Reproduction*, DOI 10.1007/978-3-319-17278-1_6

a trend towards delaying pregnancy to later in life has been observed and many women receive a diagnosis of breast cancer before completing their families [7]. In Italy, the frequency of pregnancy in women aged 35 years or more was 12 % in 1990, 16 % in 1996 and it is estimated that will amount to 25 % in 2025 [4]. Diagnosis and treatment of breast cancer often threaten fertility. Guidelines highlight the importance of discussing with patients the gonadotoxic effect of antineoplastic treatments and the risk of fertility loss as well as the available fertility preservation strategies, in addition to the chances of future conception, pregnancy and breastfeeding [8, 9].

An internet-based survey reports that more than 50 % of women at the time of diagnosis of breast cancer have fertility concerns [10], but less than 10 % of women with previous breast cancer subsequently become pregnant. This is around half the pregnancy rate seen in age-matched group without breast cancer [11]. Several studies showed that fertility counselling remains inadequate and lacks of a standardised approach [12]. The fear that pregnancy after breast cancer could worsen the prognosis does interfere with the reproductive desire of young women and impairs future conception.

There is increasing evidence in favour of the feasibility and the safety of pregnancy and breastfeeding after breast cancer; therefore, women with a history of successfully treated breast neoplasm should be given the possibility to conceive and get mother.

6.2   The Relationship Between Breast Cancer and Pregnancy

Many scientific evidences link pregnancy and risk of breast cancer. Several epidemiological studies showed a protective effect of pregnancy against breast cancer. The protection does not take place immediately: for a few years after pregnancy, there is a transient increase of breast cancer incidence. This dual effect of pregnancy on breast cancer incidence, with an increased risk for about 5–10 years after a pregnancy, followed by a lifelong protective effect, was described in a large population-based study from Norway. This study reported an increase of breast cancer incidence lasting 3 years after a full-term pregnancy, followed by long-term reduction of risk [13].

Another Norwegian registry-based study investigated the relationship between breast cancer prognosis and reproductive factors among 16,970 parous women with invasive breast tumour [14]. Analysing the relationship between parity, age and breast cancer outcome, it was observed that when diagnosis occurs before the age of 50 years, survival is worse in women with high parity compared with those with low parity. This is likely due to a combination of genetic factors, molecular characteristics of breast tumours in young patients and hormonal milieu. No clear-cut association was observed between parity and breast cancer survival when diagnosis occurs in women who were 50 years or older.

Several studies tried to explain this time-dependent effect of pregnancy on breast cancer risk. Molecular studies linked postnatal mammary involution process with susceptibility to neoplastic evolution. It is hypothesised that angiogenesis, alteration of extracellular matrix and inflammatory process are involved in this mechanism. The stroma of the mammary gland is greatly modified depending on endocrine status and reproductive factors. Post-lactational tissue remodelling may provide a break in the natural stromal barriers that suppress tumour cell motility and invasion with increased risk of tumour progression [15]. Another hypothesis involves mammary stem cells. In mouse models, it was observed that mammary stem cells are highly responsive to steroid hormone signalling, despite their ER and PgR phenotypes. Following pregnancy, it was registered a transient increase in the number of mammary stem cells, which may indicate a cellular basis for the short-term increase in breast cancer risk [16].

Pregnancy-related hormonal changes seem to be involved particularly in the long-term protective effect. Preclinical models demonstrated that high doses of estradiol induce apoptosis in long-term deprived, ER-positive breast cancer cell lines [17]. Activation of caspases via the Fas/Fal pathway appears to be involved in the promotion of apoptosis due to estradiol. The long-term oestrogen deprivation seems to sensitise breast cells to estradiol pro-apoptotic effect, with a reduction of number and growth of cancer cells in vitro. Response to estradiol depends on the ER subtypes expressed by the cells. Breast cells expressing ER-β undergo apoptosis, whereas cells expressing ER-α are protected from apoptosis. A comparative study analysed the oestrogen receptor (ER) expression in nulliparous and parous women. Compared to nulliparous women, a lower expression of ER-α and a higher expression of ER-ß was observed in parous women [18]. Other authors suggested the fetal antigen hypothesis. Clinical studies found that a high percentage of parous women, but not nulliparous women, show evidence of immunisation to antigens located on breast cancer cells. Fetal cells and breast cancer cells share common antigens: the immune response exerted by maternal immunity against fetal cells may be extended against cancer cells [19].

6.3 Pregnancy After Breast Cancer

Several case-control and population-based studies have been performed with the aim of understanding the prognostic impact of pregnancy after breast cancer. None of these studies demonstrated a negative impact of a subsequent pregnancy [20]. In particular, a meta-analysis was performed to investigate the impact of pregnancy on overall survival of women with previous breast cancer [21]. Fourteen studies were included in the meta-analysis, with a total number of 1,244 patients who became pregnant after breast cancer and 18,145 patients who did not. It was observed that women who became pregnant after adequate treatments for breast cancer had a statistically significant improvement in overall survival as compared to the control group [pooled relative risk (PRR): 0.59; confidence interval (CI): 0.50–0.70]. Analysing each study singularly, 8 studies reported a significant survival advantage for subsequent pregnancy, whilst the remaining 6 studies showed a not statistically significant trend in favour of pregnancy.

Studying the impact of pregnancy on prognosis, the "healthy mother effect" must be kept in mind. This is a relatively old concept introduced by Sankila in 1994, to explain a potential confounding factor in the interpretation of the observed effect of pregnancy in women with cancer [22]. It expresses the possibility that those women who got pregnant after breast cancer are a subgroup of patients free of relapse and healthier than the others. This could introduce a selection bias: women who become pregnant after breast cancer have better survival because they belong to a subgroup of patients with good prognosis, independently and not because of a protective effect of the pregnancy.

In the previously cited meta-analysis, a subgroup analysis in order to overcome this bias was performed. The outcome of women with pregnancy after breast cancer was compared with the outcome of controls who were known to be free of relapse. A not statistically significant trend favouring pregnancy after breast cancer was still observed [21]. Even if selection bias may partially contribute to the risk of death reduction, it seems still reasonable to conclude that pregnancy is safe in women with a history of breast cancer and does not increase the risk of recurrence.

In spite of this, a possible negative impact of pregnancy on breast cancer prognosis, particularly in patients with endocrine-responsive tumour, is still of concern. Recently, a study with the aim of investigating the effect of pregnancy in women with breast cancer according to oestrogen receptor status was conducted by Azim et al. [23]. In the three subgroups (oestrogen receptor-positive cohort, oestrogen receptor-negative cohort and all patients) no difference in disease-free survival was observed between women who become pregnant and those who did not conceive. Further, the pregnant group had better overall survival, again with no interaction observed according to ER status [23]. In summary, the study indicates that pregnancy is not protective against a relapse in patients with endocrine-sensitive tumour, but at the same time it does not exert a detrimental effect.

A further point of discussion is the time interval between the end of antineoplastic treatments and pregnancy. Several studies analysed this relationship with inconsistent results. A significant survival improvement was observed only for women who conceive after 24 months or more (Table 6.1). A not significant protection was

Table 6.1 Cox's proportional hazard model for survival in women with breast cancer with time-dependent variable stratified by time from diagnosis

Time to subsequent pregnancy (months)	Beta coefficient	P value	Hazard ratio (95 % CI)
<6	0.79	0.579	2.20 (0.14–35.42)
6–24	−0.80	0.135	0.45 (0.16–1.28)
>24	−0.74	0.009	0.48 (0.27–0.83)

(Each stratified model adjusted for age, lymph node status, and tumor size)
Modified from Ives A. et al. Pregnancy after breast cancer: population-based study. BMJ 2007;334:194

observed for women who delayed pregnancy for at least 6 months [24]. A large population-based study corroborates the theory that the risk of dying decreases with increasing the gap between diagnosis and childbirth [25].

The optimal timing of pregnancy after breast cancer is still undefined and the decision depends on patient's prognosis, age and personal condition. Because of the reassuring studies on patients who get pregnant 2 years and more after breast cancer and the observation that recurrences occur more frequently in the first few years, a delay of 2–3 years is conventionally recommended.

This time interval would also allow to recover from chemotherapy-induced ovarian toxicity. Women with ER-negative breast cancer should be advised to wait at least 6 months from the end of treatments before conceiving, to avoid the possible toxic effect of chemotherapy on growing oocytes.

As to ER-positive breast cancer, current guidelines recommend at least 5 years of endocrine therapy [26]. Furthermore, recent evidence suggests that 10 years of tamoxifen confer even greater protection [27]. Because of the teratogenetic effects of tamoxifen, pregnancy during endocrine therapy is contraindicated and an off-therapy period of 3–6 months is recommended before conceiving. But the reproductive potential is declining year by year, because of the physiological loss of ovarian reserve and the harms of chemotherapy. The feasibility of a temporary break of the hormonal therapy allowing to conceive and have a full-term pregnancy, with subsequent completion of endocrine treatment is under investigation. A prospective study of the Breast International Group and North American Breast Cancer Group (BIG-NABCG) is currently ongoing, investigating the clinical and biological features contributing to a safe and successful pregnancy in ER-positive breast cancer patients. The analysis will focus on both oncological outcomes (local and distant recurrences and survival) and obstetrical outcomes (spontaneous abortion, preterm delivery, intrauterine growth restriction, low weight at birth, fetal malformations). Secondary endpoints of the study are the feasibility and the impact of a temporary break of endocrine therapy to allow conception and the optimal duration of subsequent hormonal therapy after delivery and breastfeeding [28].

6.4   Obstetrical and Neonatal Outcome

One of the unnamed concerns that patients face is the fear of a potential teratogenic effect of antineoplastic treatments on the offspring. Few data are available on birth outcomes in breast cancer survival; however, no excess risk for the newborn health is suggested [28].

Some studies found a higher rate of abortion than in general population. This information may be biased because most of the studies did not discriminate between spontaneous and induced abortion. When this issue was considered, the risk of spontaneous abortion did not seem to be higher in breast cancer patients than in general population. On the contrary, the rate of induced abortion is consistently higher, suggesting that uncertainties of patients and physicians about safety of pregnancy after breast cancer often lead to dramatic choices [29]. Studies comparing disease-free survival in patients who completed their pregnancy to term and patients who had an abortion found a not statistically significant trend towards better outcome in women who had a full-term pregnancy [23].

Two large studies assessed the obstetrical and neonatal outcomes of pregnancies following breast cancer. A Danish nationwide cohort study investigated whether maternal breast cancer affects birth outcome [30]. Data about pregnancies of 216 women with a history of breast cancer were matched with a comparison cohort of 10,453 women belonging to general population. Similar rates of low birth weight, stillbirth and congenital abnormalities were observed in the two groups. A small and not statistically significant higher preterm delivery rate was observed in the breast cancer cohort. Mean birth weight was nearly 3,400 g in both groups, as well as mean gestational age at delivery. Different findings were reported in a Swedish cohort study aiming to assess delivery risk and neonatal health [31]. Data were extrapolated from the Swedish Medical Birth Registry and the Swedish Cancer Registry, including 331 mothers with a history of breast cancer and 2,870,518 mothers belonging to general population. An increased risk of delivery complication, caesarean section, preterm delivery and congenital malformations and no difference in low birth weight rate at delivery was observed. Authors conclusion is that pregnancy after breast cancer should be considered at high risk and therefore managed and surveilled accordingly.

Usually women with previous breast cancer are more likely to give birth at an older age than the general population. Both studies point out this difference in maternal age. About 50 % of women in breast cancer cohort are 35 years old or more at delivery, with a mean age of 34 years, whereas in the comparison group the figures are 11 % and 28 years, respectively [30, 31]. It is well known that pregnancy at an old age is more susceptible to many comorbidities and complications as gestational hypertension, preeclampsia, gestational diabetes and other conditions that bring about high risk for pregnancy outcome and require special surveillance. This may partially explain the slightly higher rate of pregnancy complications reported in the Swedish study, but uncertainties still exists.

6.5 Breastfeeding After Breast Cancer

Many factors, such as personal, cultural, social and environmental factors, influence women's decision about breastfeeding. Beyond these, breast cancer survivors face unique physical and emotional factors that might impact their decision and ability to breastfeed.

A qualitative research explored by an interview the experience and the feelings about breastfeeding in a selected group of breast cancer survivors [32]. Generally, patients alleged the wish to breastfeed, but also anxiety and concerns about doing it. This highlights the need of prenatal education and information to prepare the prospective mother to the challenges of breastfeeding. Breast cancer survivors alleged physical and emotional problems, mainly because they had to rely primarily or entirely on one breast. Treatments for breast cancer can affect lactation. Proximity of the surgical incision to the nipple-areola complex, dose and type of radiation therapy may reduce or inhibit lactation. Thus, many patients can breastfeed from the untreated breast only, with consequent uncertainty about whether or not the milk supply would be sufficient for the infant [32]. Failure to nurse from one breast should not affect the use of the other and the mother should be reassured about the adequacy of milk production by a single breast, sufficient for the nutritional need of the newborn.

Another survey analysis was performed investigating the breastfeeding patterns and habits in breast cancer survivors [33]. Hypoplasia and hypotrophia of the operated and irradiated breast were observed, with consequent reduced milk production, nipple pain, physical changes and discomfort during latching. Furthermore, a previous mastectomy was associated with short-lasting breastfeeding. This is not only justified by the fact that these patients have a single breast to nurse their babies, but also women with previous breast conserving surgery used one breast only for lactation. A possible alternative explanation is that body image plays an important role in the success of breastfeeding, and breast-conserving surgery, in spite of mastectomy, may reinforce the feeling of maternal adequacy. A proper breastfeeding counselling is a key factor for successful and prolonged breastfeeding in breast cancer survivors. This experience often brings about a psychological rehabilitation and patients express satisfaction to have been able to breastfed their babies, even if it required efforts and sometimes milk supplement.

These results enlighten the reasons of breast cancer survivors to breastfeed and the challenges which they will face and concern them. It is of the utmost importance that physicians provide practical and continuous support to the mother, especially during the postpartum period.

Beyond feasibility the safety of breastfeeding after breast cancer treatment remains an open question. Several studies have demonstrated the protective effect of breastfeeding on breast cancer risk in general population. A meta-analysis including data from 47 epidemiological studies, evaluating the relationship between breastfeeding and breast cancer, has demonstrated a 4.3 % reduction of the relative risk of breast cancer for each year that a woman breastfeeds [34]. In order to reduce biases, stratifications for age, parity, ethnicity and age at first delivery were performed, matching women who breastfed and who did not breastfeed on the basis of the same characteristics. The conclusion was that the benefits are statistically significant and breastfeeding should be encouraged.

While there is evidence that breastfeeding reduces breast cancer incidence in general population, there are no solid epidemiological data about breastfeeding after breast cancer. A retrospective case-control study investigated the survival rate of patients treated for breast cancer who subsequently became pregnant [35]. A recent re-analysis of those data was performed, specifically focused on the role of breastfeeding. A better survival was suggested in women who breastfed. These data could be biased, but it may be supposed that breastfeeding does not have a detrimental effect on breast cancer outcome [36].

The mechanisms underneath the association of breastfeeding and reduction of breast cancer incidence are not known. Several hypotheses were expressed in various studies and were synthesised in a review article [36]. Some data suggest that lactation may reduce the carcinogens level in the breast. Another hypothesis is the suckling-related blockage of the hypothalamus-pituitary axis leading to lactational amenorrhoea. From animal models, it was hypothesised that differentiation of the mammary gland as observed during pregnancy and lactation protects from neoplastic evolution. The role of prolactine has been widely studied but with conflicting results, and the impact of this hormone on initiation and promotion of breast cancer in humans remains unclear.

Epithelium changes and stromal activation which occur in remodelling breast tissue may be associated with a temporary increase in breast cancer incidence. This observation recommends a thorough follow-up of women with history of breast cancer after pregnancy or lactation. Patients and physicians often tell of the fear of a delay in diagnosis in case of tumour recurrence. Lactation does not interfere with clinical and radiological evaluation of the breasts. Ultrasound exam can be safely performed and in case of suspicion, mammography or breast magnetic resonance imaging can be performed after having drained the lactating breasts [36].

Despite uncertainty, the benefits of breastfeeding to the baby and the mother are well established. Newborns who are breastfed are protected from infections in the short period and are less susceptible to develop autoimmune diseases and metabolic disorders at adult age. Furthermore, a benefit in neurocognitive development of the baby breastfed has been suggested. Breastfeeding bears several advantages for the mother as well. Women who breastfeed have better control of postpartum bleeding, return swiftly at the usual weight and are heavily gratified by the emotional bond which is created with her baby.

In conclusion, current evidence suggests that breast cancer survivors who wish to breastfeed, should be encouraged and supported in their efforts.

6.6   Childbearing Attitudes of Young Breast Cancer Survivors

Many studies have shown that pregnancy and parenthood are two important issues for young women with breast cancer. As breast cancer-related mortality declines, the impact of anticancer treatments on reproductive potential is getting more relevant, and fertility impairment may worsen the quality of life in a growing number of patients. For some young breast cancer survivors, the threat to their childbearing plans has major emotional and psychological consequences. Literature and clinical practice demonstrate that some women remain fertile and have a spontaneous pregnancy after a history of cancer. Additionally, the advent of advanced assisted reproductive technology within the oncology field has made fertility preservation an option for women, prior to the initiation of treatments. As known, other options are available for infertile women, such as adoption and third-party reproduction, but most couples crave biological offspring.

Several studies showed that the risk of early menopause and infertility are causes of concern for about the half of young women who receive breast cancer diagnosis. Some patients reported that this fear conditioned treatment decisions [37]. Infertility in cancer patients is associated, more frequently than in general population, to anxiety, depressive symptoms and sexual impairment which have a negative impact on the quality of life.

But even when fertility is preserved, other concerns upset breast cancer patients. Women fear that the child might be born with a birth defect because of the chemotherapeutic agents they received. They are anxious about a shorter life expectancy and are afraid of having not enough energies to raise children. Furthermore, women feared that the offspring would have a greater susceptibility to cancer [38].

On the other hand, some patients perceive the benefits that could be achieved by having children after breast cancer treatment. Raising a child can be a powerful motivator to stay alive and healthy, it may strengthen the relationship with the partner, it brings back normalcy in their life and it would restore the sense of femininity and sexuality [39]. Breast cancer survivors who are disease-free often feel healthy enough to consider a pregnancy. This is called a reasonable wellness, which may express the ethical guide into the difficult choice of getting mother.

In clinical practice, gynaecologists and oncologists are frequently faced with the issue of educating women about childbearing after breast cancer. However, some studies suggested that these professionals often feel discomfort and lack of knowledge about how to best educate women with cancer-related fertility matters, leaving women's fertility concerns poorly addressed. Attending physicians may perceive the fertility preservation as a low priority issue, compared with the treatment of cancer or they could fear that fertility preservation techniques may dwindle the efficacy of anticancer treatments. Presently, there are guidelines stressing the need to communicate with and educate young patients regarding fertility issues. Oncologists should refer interested and appropriate patients to reproductive specialists as early as possible, to allow a rapid access to fertility preservation strategies and to avoid delaying the chemotherapy onset [8, 9].

6.7   Breast Cancer, Pregnancy and Breastfeeding in BRCA1/2 Mutation Carriers

Reproductive factors influence the risk of breast cancer in the general population, but few data are available in the selected group of women with mutations in BRCA1 and BRCA2 genes. BRCA1 and BRCA2 are tumour suppressor genes which are involved in multiple processes, including DNA damage repair and recombination, and regulate normal cell differentiation. During pregnancy and breastfeeding, breast cells divide and differentiate; thus, it could be supposed that reproductive factors have different impacts on breast cancer risk in the BRCA mutation carriers and in general population.

A large retrospective cohort study including women carrying BRCA1/2 mutations investigated the impact of pregnancy on breast cancer incidence [40]. No difference was found between parous and nulliparous women, and the same results were observed in BRCA1 and BRCA2 mutation carriers. It does not appear that parity per se influences the risk of breast cancer in this particular subgroup of women.

Inconsistent results are reported about the association between breastfeeding and breast cancer risk. Some evidences suggest a protective effects of breastfeeding, even stronger than in general population, but only among BRCA1 mutation carriers [41, 42].

It is known that hereditary breast cancer is different from sporadic tumour and differences are observed between breast cancer patients with BRCA1 and BRCA2 mutations as well. This might suggest that the biological pathway for carcinogenesis is different for these two genes.

Our knowledge about the impact of pregnancy after breast cancer in BRCA1/2 mutation carriers is even poorer. This is partly due to the small proportion of women carrying mutations in these genes. The question is sensible, because of the typical early age of onset of hereditary breast cancer. A multicenter, case-control study which included women known to carry a BRCA 1 or BRCA 2 mutation and history of breast cancer has been published recently [43]. The cases were patients with pregnancy-associated breast cancer or pregnancy following breast cancer. The controls were selected among patients who did not get pregnant after breast cancer diagnosis and who were alive and recurrence-free at the time of the delivery of the baby in the matched group, in order to reduce potential confounding bias, such as the healthy mother effect. The 15-year survival was excellent in the two groups, around 90 %, and no significant difference was observed between cases and controls after adjustment for several prognostic factors. Despite the limitations of the study, first of all the small sample size, these results are encouraging and future research is recommended to prove the not detrimental effect of pregnancy after breast cancer in this particular subgroup of women [43].

There is an issue in BRCA1/2 mutation carriers that deserves special consideration. Some studies suggested that the deficient DNA repair mechanism due to mutations in BRCA 1 and BRCA 2 genes may make oocytes more susceptible to DNA-damaging agents. Furthermore, it has been speculated that BRCA mutation carriers may have a lesser ovarian reserve than general population and undergo premature menopause. As a consequence, BRCA mutation carriers may be more susceptible to chemotherapy-induced gonadotoxicity with severe ovarian reserve loss [44]. Diagnosis of breast cancer in a young patient with BRCA mutation raises concerns about her future fertility. A trend towards earlier referral to fertility specialists underscores the importance of this issue. However, the better approach in this particular group of patients is not an easy choice. On one side data suggest a poor response to ovarian stimulation for oocyte retrieval and cryopreservation, particularly in BRCA1 mutation carriers; on the other side ovarian tissue cryopreservation for BRCA mutation carrier is disputed because of the risk of ovarian cancer and lastly the efficacy of temporary ovarian suppression with GnRH agonists is still controversial [44].

All these findings suggest that BRCA mutation carriers may have a shorter reproductive life, and this should be taken into account in the management of young breast cancer patients who desire a future pregnancy. Whether or not the low ovarian reserve and poor response to ovarian stimulation may reduce the fertility potential of women with BRCA mutations is still unknown and further research is needed.

References

1. De Angelis R, Sant M, Coleman MP, et al. Cancer survival in Europe 1999-2007 by country and age: results of EUROCARE-5-a population-based study. Lancet Oncol. 2014;15(1): 23–34.
2. Coleman MP, Quaresma M, Berrino F, et al. Cancer survival in five continents: a worldwide population-based study (CONCORD). Lancet Oncol. 2008;9(8):730–56.
3. Jemal A, Bray F, Center MM, et al. Global cancer statistics. Cancer J Clin. 2011;61(2):69–90.
4. Linee guida AIOM. Preservazione della fertilità nei pazienti oncologici. Edizione 2013. http://www.aiom.it/.
5. Azim HA, Michiels S, Bedard P, et al. Elucidating prognosis and biology of breast cancer arising in young women using gene expression profiling. Clin Cancer Res. 2012;18(5):1341–51.
6. Fredholm H, Eaker S, Frisell J, et al. Breast cancer in young women: poor survival despite intensive treatment. PLoS One. 2009;4(11):e7695.
7. Berkowitz GS, Skovron ML, Lapinski RH, et al. Delayed childbearing and the outcome of pregnancy. N Engl J Med. 1990;322(10):659–64.
8. Lee SJ, Schover LR, Partridge AH, et al. American Society of Clinical Oncology recommendations on fertility preservation in cancer patients. J Clin Oncol. 2006;24(18):2917–31.
9. Loren AW, Mangu PB, Nohr Beck L, et al. Fertility preservation for patients with cancer: American Society of Clinical Oncology clinical practice guideline update. J Clin Oncol. 2013;31(19):2500–10.
10. Partridge AH, Gelber S, Peppercorn J, et al. Web-based survey of fertility issues in young women with breast cancer. J Clin Oncol. 2004;22(20):4174–83.
11. Pagani O, Azim HA. Pregnancy after breast cancer: myths and facts. Breast Cancer. 2012;7:210–4.
12. Peccatori FA, Azim HA. Pregnancy in breast cancer survivors: a need for proper counselling. Breast. 2009;18(6):337–8.
13. Albrektsen G, Heuch I, Hansen S, et al. Breast cancer risk by age at birth, time since birth and time intervals between births: exploring interaction effects. Br J Cancer. 2005;92(1):167–75.
14. Alsaker MDK, Opdahl S, Romundstad PR, et al. Association of time since last birth, age at first birth and parity with breast cancer survival among parous women: a register-based study from Norway. Int J Cancer. 2013;132:174–81.
15. Bemis LT, Schedin P. Reproductive state of rat mammary gland stroma modulates human breast cancer cell migration and invasion. Cancer Res. 2000;60(13):3414–8.
16. Asselin-Labat ML, Vaillant F, Sheridan JM, et al. Control of mammary stem cell function by steroid hormone signalling. Nature. 2010;465(7299):798–802.
17. Song RX, Mor G, Naftolin F, et al. Effect of long term estrogen deprivation on apoptotic responses of breast cancer cells to 17β-estradiol. J Natl Cancer Inst. 2001;93(22):1714–23.
18. Asztalos S, Gann PH, Hayes MK, et al. Gene expression patterns in the human breast after pregnancy. Cancer Prev Res. 2010;3(3):301–11.
19. Janerich DT. The fetal antigen hypothesis: cancer and beyond. Med Hypotheses. 2001; 56(1):101–3.
20. Azim HA, Peccatori FA, de Ezambuja E, et al. Motherhood after breast cancer: searching for la dolce vita. Expert Rev Anticancer Ther. 2011;11(2):287–98.
21. Azim HA, Santoro L, Pavlidis N, et al. Safety of pregnancy following breast cancer diagnosis: a meta-analysis of 14 studies. Eur J Cancer. 2011;47:74–83.
22. Sankila R, Heinavaara S, Hakulinen T, et al. Survival of breast cancer patients after subsequent term pregnancy: "healthy mother effect". Am J Obstet Gynecol. 1994;170(3):818–23.
23. Azim HA, Kroman N, Paesmans M, et al. Prognostic impact of pregnancy after breast cancer according to estrogen receptor status: a multicentre retrospective study. J Clin Oncol. 2013; 31(1):73–9.
24. Ives A, Saunders C, Bulsara M, et al. Pregnancy after breast cancer: population based study. BMJ. 2007;334:194.
25. Verkooijen HM, Lim GH, Czene K, et al. Effect of childbirth after treatment on long-term survival from breast cancer. Br J Surg. 2010;97(8):1253–9.

26. Cardoso F, Loibl S, Pagani O, et al. The European Society of Breast Cancer Specialists recommendations for the management of young women with breast cancer. Eur J Cancer. 2012;48(18):3355–77.
27. Davies C, Pan H, Godwin J, et al. Long-term effects of continuing adjuvant tamoxifen to 10 years versus stopping at 5 years after diagnosis of oestrogen receptor-positive breast cancer: ATLAS, a randomised trial. Lancet. 2013;381:805–16.
28. Pagani O, Partridge A, Korde L, et al. Pregnancy after breast cancer: if you wish, ma'am. Breast Cancer Res Treat. 2011;129:309–17.
29. Kroman N, Jensen MB, Wohlfahrt J, et al. Pregnancy after treatment of breast cancer – a population-based study on behalf of Danish Breast Cancer Cooperative Group. Acta Oncol. 2008;47(4):545–9.
30. Langagergaard V, Gislum M, Skriver MV, et al. Birth outcome in women with breast cancer. Br J Cancer. 2006;94:142–6.
31. Dalberg K, Eriksson J, Holmberg L. Birth outcome in women with previously treated breast cancer – A population-based cohort study from Sweden. PLoS One. 2006;3(9):e336.
32. Gorman JR, Usita PM, Madlensky L, et al. A qualitative investigation of breast cancer survivors' experiences with breastfeeding. J Cancer Surviv. 2009;3:181–91.
33. Azim HA, Bellettini G, Liptrott SJ, et al. Breastfeeding in breast cancer survivors: pattern, behaviour and effect on breast cancer outcome. Breast. 2010;19:527–31.
34. Collaborative Group on Hormonal Factors in Breast Cancer. Breast cancer and breastfeeding: collaborative reanalysis of individual data from 47 epidemiological studies in 30 countries, including 50302 women with breast cancer and 96973 women without the disease. Lancet. 2002;360(9328):187–95.
35. Gelber S, Coates AS, Goldhirsch A, et al. Effect of pregnancy on overall survival after the diagnosis of early stage breast cancer. J Clin Oncol. 2001;19:1671–5.
36. Azim HA, Bellettini G, Gelber S, et al. Breast-feeding after breast cancer: if you wish, madam. Breast Cancer Res Treat. 2009;114:7–12.
37. Ruddy KJ, Gelber SI, Tamimi RM, et al. Prospective study of fertility concerns and preservation strategies in young women with breast cancer. J Clin Oncol. 2014;32(11):1151–6.
38. Fossa SD, Magelssen H, Melve K, et al. Parenthood in survivors after adulthood cancer and perinatal health in their offspring: a preliminary report. J Natl Cancer Inst Monogr. 2005;34: 77–82.
39. Goncalves V, Sehovic I, Quinn G. Childbearing attitudes and decisions of young breast cancer survivors: a systematic review. Hum Reprod Update. 2014;20(2):279–92.
40. Andrieu N, Goldgar DE, Easton DF, et al. Pregnancies, breast-feeding and breast cancer risk in the International BRCA1/2 Carrier Cohort Study (IBCCS). J Natl Cancer Inst. 2006; 98(8):535–44.
41. Kotsopoulos J, Lubinski J, Salmena L, et al. Breastfeeding and the risk of breast cancer in BRCA 1 and BRCA2 mutation carriers. Breast Cancer Res. 2012;14:R42.
42. Jernstrom H, Lubinski H, Lynch T, et al. Breast-feeding and the risk of breast cancer in BRCA1 and BRCA2 mutation carriers. J Natl Cancer Inst. 2004;96(14):1094–8.
43. Valentini A, Lubinski J, Byrski T, et al. The impact of pregnancy on breast cancer survival in women who carry a BRCA1 or BRCA2 mutation. Breast Cancer Res Treat. 2013;142:177–85.
44. Rodriguez-Wallberg KA, Oktay K. Fertility preservation and pregnancy in women with and without BRCA mutation positive breast cancer. Oncologist. 2012;17:1409–17.

Reproductive Issues in BRCA Mutation Carriers

Shani Paluch-Shimon, Dror Meirow, and Jordana Hyman

7.1 BRCA1/2 Mutations and Breast Cancer: Introduction

7.1.1 Background

While the majority of cancer cases occur sporadically with no evident family history of cancer in immediate family members, in a subset of cases, estimated at 5–10 % of incident cancers, a strong inherited predisposition is noted [1, 2]. Clinically, phenotypic features such as familial, cross-generational clustering of cancer, early age at diagnosis compared with the average risk population, and syndromic association between cancers have been applied as indicators hallmarking cancer predisposition [3].

7.1.2 BRCA1/2 and Cancer Risk

A germline mutation in either the *BRCA1* (MIM# 113705) or the *BRCA2* (MIM # 600185) genes is the most significant known risk factor (other than gender and

S. Paluch-Shimon (✉)
Breast Cancer Service for Young Women, Breast Oncology Institute,
Tel Hashomer 52621, Israel

Division of Oncology, Sheba Medical Centre, Tel Hashomer 52621, Israel
e-mail: Shani.paluch-shimon@sheba.health.gov.il

D. Meirow
Fertility Preservation, IVF Unit, Department of Obstetrics & Gynaecology,
Sheba Medical Centre, Tel Hashomer 52621, Israel
e-mail: Dror.meirow@sheba.health.gov.il

J. Hyman
IVF Unit, Department of Obstetrics and Gynecology, The Hadassah University
Hospital, Ein Kerem, Jerusalem, Israel
e-mail: jordana@hadassah.org.il

© Springer International Publishing Switzerland 2015
N. Biglia, F.A. Peccatori (eds.), *Breast Cancer, Fertility Preservation and Reproduction*, DOI 10.1007/978-3-319-17278-1_7

increasing age) for developing breast and ovarian cancer. Mutations in these genes are highly penetrant and confer a lifetime risk of developing breast cancer (BC) of 40–90 % and up to a 60 % lifetime risk of developing ovarian cancer [4–9]. The biological rationale and proposed molecular mechanism that underlies the elevated risk for cancer are that *BRCA1* and *BRCA2* proteins play a pivotal role in DNA repair mechanisms. Specifically, *BRCA1* and *BRCA2* are critical in the repair of double-stranded DNA breaks via homologous recombination and for maintaining genomic stability [10, 11]. A deficiency in a cell's ability to repair DNA damage increases genomic instability which in turn can increase the risk of initiating carcinogenesis. Unlike other environmental and lifestyle risk factors for BC, distinct phenotypic characteristics of *BRCA1/2*-associated BCs have been described. Thus *BRCA1/2* plays not only an important role on the causal pathway for developing BC, but also has a significant impact on the biological and clinical characteristics of *BRCA1/2*-associated BCs.

In unselected groups of young BC patients, a *BRCA1/2* mutation was prevalent in 9 % of women under 39 years of age in a study by Golshan et al. and in 5.9 % of women under 36 years of age in a study by Peto et al. [12, 13]. In selected groups of young Ashkenazi Jewish (AJ) women with BC, *BRCA1/2* mutations were noted in 8–20 % [14, 15]. Noteworthy, the mutational spectrum of germline mutations in this genetically homogeneous population is limited to three germline mutations in *BRCA1* (185delAG, 5382insC) and *BRCA2* (6174delT) accounting for the majority of high-risk families [16].

7.1.3 Counseling

Until both BRCA genes were cloned, cancer-free family members of high-risk families were counseled regarding their lifetime risk of being diagnosed with cancer, based on the cancer phenotype in their family. Recommendations for early detection and prevention were also dictated by the familial cancer phenotype. Over the past 20 years, cloning of *BRCA1/2* in hereditary breast/ovarian cancer has enhanced cancer genetics services, enabling objective assessment of cancer risk by genetically testing high-risk individuals. Cancer risk evaluation and clear guidelines and recommendations including early detection schemes and/or risk-reducing surgeries are now based on the genotype, rather than the phenotype. Furthermore, genotypic-based risk assessment has enabled clinicians to reassure family members found not to harbor the familial mutation, and to reinstate average cancer risk status. There are extensive guidelines for genetic testing and risk assessment in addition to guidelines for BC risk reduction and early detection schemes and ovarian cancer screening; however, these are beyond the scope of this chapter (refer Table 7.1). One of the most important factors relevant to this chapter is ovarian cancer risk reduction – with the universal recommendation for bilateral risk-reducing salpingo-oophorectomy (RRSO) for women harboring a *BRCA1/2* mutation, between 35 and 40 years of age either after completion of childbearing, or individualized based on family history of earliest onset case of ovarian cancer. RRSO has consistently

Table 7.1 NCCN Guidelines recommend that BRCA1/2 testing be performed for an individual with a history of breast cancer at least and one of the following criteria [22]

Diagnosed at or before 45 years of age
Having 2 breast primaries with one being diagnosed ≤50 years of age
Diagnosed ≤50 years with at least 1 close relative with a breast cancer diagnosis
Diagnosed with triple negative breast cancer at ≤60 years
Diagnosed at any age with at least 1 close relative with a breast cancer diagnosis at ≤50 years
Diagnosed at any age with 2 or more close relatives with a breast cancer diagnosis at any age or with ≥1 close relative diagnosed with epithelial ovarian cancer at any age
Diagnosed at any age with at 2 or more close relatives with pancreatic cancer or aggressive prostate cancer at any age
Having a close male relative with breast cancer at any age
Ashkenazi Jewish ethnicity

demonstrated a dramatic reduction in the risk of developing ovarian and fallopian tube cancer by over 80–85 % [17, 18] although a residual risk for primary peritoneal cancer of 1–4.3 % remains [17–20]. Furthermore, RRSO performed before 40 years of age has been demonstrated to reduce early onset BC risk by approximately 50 % [20, 21]. Consideration of reproductive desires of women is important in designating the timing of RRSO, and women need to be counseled about the consequences of premature menopause.

7.1.4 Clinicopathologic Characteristics and Prognosis

BRCA1- and *BRCA2*-associated BCs are often diagnosed at an earlier age and at a later stage [23]. Due to elevated breast density, BRCA1/2-associated BCs are also less likely to be detected by mammography and ultrasound screening in young women, and tumors with "pushing margins" are less visible on mammography [24]. *BRCA1*-associated tumors are more likely to have high histological grade, lack estrogen and progesterone receptors, lack HER2/neu over-expression, and be of triple negative (TN) and medullary subtypes [25–27]. All these factors have an impact on diagnosis and treatment decisions - patients with high grade, endocrine unresponsive tumors more likely to receive chemotherapy.

Several studies have focused on whether prognosis and outcome differ between BRCA-associated BC compared with those in noncarriers. Retrospective studies by Rennert et al. [28] and Huzarski and coworkers both reported no difference in 10-year survival in patients with *BRCA1* mutations compared to those without mutations [29]. Several smaller studies reported similar results [25, 30]. Goodwin et al. corroborate these findings, reporting no discernible overall survival benefit among *BRCA1* or *BRCA2* breast cancer mutation carriers who received adjuvant chemotherapy ($n = 164$) compared to non-BRCA controls ($n = 1,550$) [31]. Furthermore, studies that focused on TN BCs also reported no difference in outcome between *BRCA1/BRCA2* positive and non-*BRCA1/BRCA2* TN cases [32, 33].

7.1.5   Treatment of *BRCA1/2*-Associated Breast Cancer

Importantly, *BRCA1/BRCA2* deficient cells are considered to be more sensitive to chemotherapy because of the underlying deficiency in double-stranded DNA repair [34–36]. Specifically, preclinical models suggested that *BRCA* mutant cells were more sensitive to chemotherapy that cause double-strand breaks in DNA, such as platinum compounds, anthracyclines, and alkylators [37–40]. When assessing the clinical response of *BRCA1/2*-mutated breast cancers to therapy, differential response to certain chemotherapy drugs had been proposed [41–43]. Thus, it was suggested that *BRCA1* deficient tumors may be more responsive to platinum compounds [44–46] and less responsive to taxanes [41, 47–49]. Byrski et al. reported pathological complete responses to neo-adjuvant cisplatinum as high as 83 % (10/12) in *BRCA1* carriers [44, 48]. *BRCA1/BRCA2*-associated cancers are eligible for targeted biological therapies by PARP (poly-ADP-ribose polymerase) inhibitors that specifically target the DNA repair pathway in *BRCA1/BRCA2* deficient cells [36, 50]. Poly (ADP-ribose) polymerase1 (PARP1) plays a key role in the repair of DNA single-strand breaks through base excision repair. The inhibition of PARP1 leads to the accumulation of single-strand breaks in DNA and consequently to double-strand breaks at the replication forks. Normally, these double-strand breaks are repaired by homologous recombination (HR). However, when cancer cells deficient of HR due to absent *BRCA* are exposed to PARP1 inhibitors they accumulate unrepaired double-strand breaks that result in collapse of the replication forks and cell death. Such synergistic cell death resulting from concomitant inhibition of molecular pathways that are each dispensable when inactivated solely is a concept known as "synthetic lethality." Since the normal cells of *BRCA* mutation carriers contain one functional allele of *BRCA*, they can still use HR and repair DSB, and therefore they are resistant to PARP inhibition. Thus, PARP inhibitors selectively target only the cancer cells and are associated with relatively minor damage to the normal tissues [35]. In recent years, several potent PARP inhibitors were developed and evaluated, alone and in combination with chemotherapy, for the treatment of *BRCA*-mutated cancers. The pivotal trial assessing PARP inhibitors in a study population enriched for *BRCA* mutation carriers was published by Fong et al. [51]. Evidence of sustained antitumor activity was limited to patients with *BRCA-associated* cancers, of whom 63 % experienced clinical benefit. A proof-of-concept study evaluating Olaparib in *BRCA*-associated advanced BC was next published by Tutt et al. [52]. The first adjuvant trial assessing use of PARP inhibitors in *BRCA1/2*-associated BC named OLYMPIA opened in 2014, comparing 12 months of adjuvant Olaparib versus placebo following completion of standard neo-adjuvant/adjuvant chemotherapy. The impact of PARP inhibitors on ovarian function is currently unknown.

7.2   Hormonal Contraception in BRCA Mutation Carriers

Hormonal contraception in women with BC is controversial, specifically in BRCA carriers, due to both potential benefits and risks [53]. The literature has focused on the oral contraceptive pill (OCP); however, other forms of hormonal contraception are also debatable.

There is evidence that levonorgestrel-releasing intrauterine system (LNG-IUS) may be effective in protecting the endometrium in women with BC, after tamoxifen therapy [54–56]. Benefits include reduced endometrial hyperplasia and endometrial polyps. Most studies found no evidence of increased BC recurrence or cancer-related deaths in women who used LNG-IUS; however, in one Belgian study, there was an increase in cancer recurrence rate in women diagnosed with BC while using LNG-IUS and continuing to use the device [57]. Another study found a small increased risk of BC recurrence [58]. No studies specifically address BRCA mutation carriers and LNG-IUS.

While until now RRSO has been the gold standard for ovarian cancer risk reduction in this population, more recently, prophylactic bilateral salpingectomy, followed by delayed oophorectomy close to menopause, has been proposed as an alternative approach to reduce ovarian cancer risk [59, 60]. This is yet to be evaluated in a clinical trial setting. Women who are still considering reproduction, or who do not wish to undergo surgical prevention, may be candidates for OCP use in reducing ovarian cancer risk.

The recent long-term follow-up of OCP use in the Nurses Health study [61] demonstrated a trend towards increased premature mortality due to BC (test for trend $p < 0.0001$) and decreased mortality rates due to ovarian cancer ($p = 0.0020$) in women who had used OCP. A cohort study of Jewish BRCA1 and BRCA2 mutation carriers [62] showed a significantly increased risk of early onset BC in women who had used the OCP, with average age of onset 6 years earlier than nonusers.

A meta-analysis of studies examining OCP use and BC risk found that although there was a significant increase in BC in women with BRCA mutations in cohort studies, no significantly increased risk was demonstrated in case-control studies [63]. The same analysis showed a significant reduction in the risk of ovarian cancer associated with OCP use. Their conclusion was that OCP may be considered as an alternative to RRSO for prevention of ovarian cancer in women with BRCA1 mutation, although this has not been adopted as a standard practice.

Age of OCP use appears to be important in BC risk. There is evidence that teenage (<20 years) [64] or young adult (<25) [65] OCP use may increase the risk of BC in women with BRCA mutations, especially BRCA1. Other studies demonstrated increased risk in BRCA1 mutation carriers who used the OCP prior to age 30 [66].

The dose of estradiol in the OCP, and the actual formulation, may also be relevant in BC risk. OCP use prior to 1975 (higher dose estrogen) increases the risk of BC in BRCA mutation carriers [67, 68].

Several studies show a small or modest increase in BC risk with OCP use [67, 69, 70], while others show no increased risk with low-dose OCP [71–73]. In BRCA2 carriers, specifically, there appears to be no risk [67]. A meta-analysis of 18 studies assessing association between OCP use and breast and ovarian cancer in women carrying BRCA1/2 mutations [68] demonstrated significantly reduced risk of ovarian cancer and no increased risk in BC with newer OCPs.

Duration of OCP use may be associated with BC risk, with increased risk demonstrated for over 5 years of use [67]. Kostopolous [65] showed increased risk for each year of use when OCP was commenced prior to age 20. A meta-analysis showed no consistent trends of increasing risk with longer duration use of OCP for either BRCA1 or BRCA2 carriers [69].

A recent meta-analysis [69] found that the association between OCP use and ovarian and breast cancer risk in women with BRCA mutation were comparable to risks in the general population, with a nonstatistically significant association with BC, and inverse association with ovarian cancer.

Healthy Women carrying BRCA1 and BRCA2 mutations should be carefully counseled regarding OCP use. Younger women specifically, aged less than 30, should be aware of the potential additional risks of early onset BC. Women aged 30 years and older, who are not yet ready for RRSO, and who are desiring contraception, may be cautiously offered OCP, after discussion of risks and benefits.

7.3   Parity and Breastfeeding in BRCA Carriers

7.3.1   Age at Menarche

Younger age at menarche is associated with increased risk for sporadic early onset BC [74, 75]. An effect was not observed in BRCA2 carriers, but BRCA1 carriers whose age at menarche was 14–15 years had a 54 % reduction in BC risk compared to those with menarche at ≤ 11 years of age (OR=0.46; 95 % CI 0.30–0.69) [76].

7.3.2   Parity

Increasing parity and breastfeeding have been demonstrated to be protective against BC, but the magnitude of this protection seems to be lesser so for women with early onset BC [77, 78]. In BRCA1 and BRCA2 carriers, parity effects may also be age dependent. While an early report suggested that parity may increase risk for early onset (<40 year) BC in BRCA1 carriers [79], a larger retrospective study of 1,260 carrier pairs by the same group did not confirm this finding, and even observed decreased BC risk in BRCA1 carriers with ≥ 4 children (OR=0.62; 95 CI 0.41–0.94, vs. nulliparous carriers) [80]. In BRCA2 carriers, this study found that parity caused a borderline increase in risk for BC before age 50 (OR = 1.17 for each pregnancy; 95 CI 1.01–1.36) [80]. In a case-only study, young age at first pregnancy delayed onset of BC in carriers [8], and a retrospective study of 1,601 carriers found that in women over 40, each full-term pregnancy reduced BC risk by 14 % (95 CI 6–22 %). An age effect was seen in BRCA2 carriers with later first pregnancies associated with increased risk, whereas BRCA1 carriers with first birth over age 30 were at lower risk than those with first birth before age 20 [81]. In a case-control study by Antoniou et al, parous *BRCA1* and *BRCA2* mutation carriers were at a significantly lower risk of developing BC (hazard ratio 0.54, 95 % confidence interval 0.37–0.81) and yet the protective effect was observed only among carriers who were older than 40 years. Increasing age at first live birth was associated with an increased BC risk among *BRCA2* mutation carriers but not *BRCA1* carriers [82]. Yet other studies have failed to demonstrate an association between BC risk and age at first birth among mutation carriers [83]. A meta-analysis by Pan et al. demonstrated no association between parity and BC risk in women harboring a BRCA1/2 mutation and late age at first birth was found to be protective among BRCA1 mutation carriers [84]. These results were supported by a meta-analysis by Friebel et al. [53]. A study by Lecarpentier et al. suggests that the impact of parity on reducing BC risk in BRCA1 mutation carriers is limited to those with a mutation in the central region of BRCA1 [85].

7.3.3 Breastfeeding

In a case-control study of 965 BRCA1 and 280 BRCA2 pairs, breastfeeding did not influence BC risk in BRCA2 carriers, but BRCA1 carriers who breastfed for over 1 year were less likely to have had BC than those who never breastfed (OR = 0.55; 95 CI 0.38–0.80) [86]. A retrospective cohort study of 1,601 carriers did not show any breastfeeding effect (HR = 0.89 ,95 CI 0.62–1.27) [81]. A case-control study of 1,665 pairs demonstrated a protective effect of breastfeeding for BRCA1 carriers only, with the protective effect increasing with increasing duration of breastfeeding – a 32 % risk reduction for 1 year (OR = 0.68; 95 % CI 0.52–0.91) and 49 % risk reduction (OR = 0.51; 95 % CI 0.35–0.74) for greater than 2 years of breastfeeding [87]. In a meta-analysis by Pan et al. among BRCA1 mutation carriers, only breastfeeding for at least 1 or 2 years was associated with a 37 % reduction in BC risk (RR = 0.63, 95 % CI = 0.46–0.86) [84].

7.4 Ovarian Reserve and Infertility in BRCA Carriers

BRCA1 and BRCA2 mutation carriers conventionally undergo RRSO at the completion of childbearing, in order to reduce their risk of both ovarian and breast cancer [88]. These women experience induced surgical menopause, and thus determination of their expected fertility or ovarian reserve, or assessment of early menopause, is not possible. However, it has been hypothesized that BRCA mutations, in particular BRCA1, may be associated with reduced fertility. This is expressed by increased chemotherapy-induced amenorrhea [89], premature menopause [90–93], primary occult ovarian insufficiency [94], reduced ovarian reserve [95], and infertility [96–98].

The proposed link between BRCA mutation and fertility is suggested by several possible theories. BRCA 1 is a tumor suppressor, associated with telomere length [99, 100]. It is important in maintaining stability of the genome, as well as playing a role in DNA repair [101, 102]. BRCA1 may also have a role in protecting cells against oxidative stress [103]. Mutations in BRCA1 may lead to compromised genome integrity and deficiencies in double-stranded DNA repair [10]. Primordial follicles may be particularly sensitive to incidental DNA damage. Accumulation of DNA damage then results in oocyte apoptosis. This is turn would cause reduced ovarian reserve, decreased fertility, and earlier menopause.

Titus et al. [104] analyzed expression of DNA repair genes in human oocytes, including BRCA1. They proposed that in women with BRCA1 mutation, two processes occur concurrently during reproductive aging. As the DNA repair efficiency undergoes natural decline, double-stranded DNA breaks (DSDs) accumulate and thus more oocytes undergo apoptosis. In women with BRCA1 mutations, oocyte aneuploidy is augmented, probably due to reduced function of BRCA1 and resultant accumulation of DSDs, as well as other possible effects of BRCA1 mutation. The age-related decline in BRCA1 carriers is thus linked to earlier menopause, diminished ovarian reserve, and increased vulnerability to chemotherapy-induced amenorrhea [98]. This decline may be not be clinically apparent before age 35, when the age-related decline becomes more important.

BRCA1 appears to be upregulated in human male and female germ cells and in preimplantation embryos [105], which may support another possible mechanism involving BRCA1 dysfunction and altered human embryogenesis.

A potential link between BRCA mutation and FMR1 mutation, which is known to be associated with primary ovarian insufficiency [106] has also been proposed, suggesting that the diminished ovarian reserve in women with BRCA mutations may be FMR1 mediated. An initial study revealed a different distribution of constitutional FMR1 genotypes in BRCA mutation carriers compared with female controls [90]. BRCA mutation carriers almost uniformly expressed het-norm/low FMR1 sub-genotype. The same study group showed a trend towards earlier menopause in the BRCA1/2 carriers [90]. A subsequent study [107] found no association between low FMR1 sub-genotypes and BRCA1 mutation carriers.

7.5 Premature Menopause

Menopause is defined as commencing 12 months after the last menstrual period. Menopause occurs when the remaining follicle count reaches 1,000 or below. The years preceding menopause represent the decreasing number of follicles, but also reduced quality of oocytes, with increased risk of aneuploidy, increased risk of spontaneous miscarriage, and infertility. Evidence of earlier menopause in BRCA mutation carriers would imply reduced fertility at an earlier age, with lower ovarian reserve.

Age at menopause is multifactorial, and includes hereditary and environmental factors, including smoking. Ninety percent of women undergo menopause between the ages of 45–55, average age 51 [108]. Premature menopause, or primary ovarian insufficiency, which occurs in approximately 1 % of women, has a strong hereditary component, with over 15 % having a first-degree relative with premature menopause [109]. The commonest genetic causes are Fragile X mutation, with a mutation of the FMR1 gene, and Turner syndrome (monosomy X). Premature menopause can also be associated with autoimmune disease. Iatrogenic causes include gonadotoxic chemotherapy and radiotherapy, and surgical menopause.

Several studies have compared age at menopause between BRCA carriers and various control groups. Lin et al. [93] assessed age at natural menopause in women who were BRCA mutation carriers and women in the general population in San Francisco.

Risks were adjusted for known risk factors including smoking, oral contraceptive use, and parity. The median age at the time of natural menopause in the BRCA1/2 carriers was significantly younger than in controls (50 years vs 53 years; $p < 0.001$). In women defined as current heavy smokers (more than 1 pack per day), the median age was 46 in BRCA carriers compared with 49 in controls ($p < 0.027$). No difference in age was observed in BRCA 1 and BRCA 2 carriers.

A recent large study compared the rate of premature menopause in BRCA mutation carriers and age-matched controls who were not carriers. Controls were either family members of known mutation carriers who tested negative, or women with a family or personal history of breast or ovarian cancer, who were found not to be carriers of known mutations. There were no significant differences between the groups for parity, age at first birth, or age at last birth. Age at menopause was significantly younger in BRCA mutation carriers (49.0 vs. 50.3 years; $p < 0.001$). The difference was also observed for both BRCA1 (48.8 vs. 49.9 years; $p < 0.06$) and BRCA 2 carriers (49.2 vs. 50.8 years; $p < 0.006$). Twelve women (4.7 %) with a BRCA mutation experienced menopause before age 40 compared with three women (1.4 %) in the control group ($p < 0.04$). The observed rate of premature menopause, which is defined as menopause before age 40, is 1 % [110]. There were no differences in reported fertility problems or use of fertility medications.

Collins et al. [111] analyzed BRCA mutation carriers ($n = 829$) and family members who were negative for BRCA mutation ($n = 1,021$), for the risk of natural menopause at given ages. They included covariates of smoking, BMI, parity, age at first birth, alcohol, and fertility medications. Nineteen percent of women in the study had undergone menopause; however, no difference was observed for age-specific incidence of natural menopause between BRCA mutation carriers and noncarriers.

A study of ovarian morphology in postmenopausal women who underwent oophorectomy, assessed "signs of estrogenization" as part of the histopathological examination, in women with and without BRCA1 mutation [112]. Women with BRCA1 mutation had absent signs of estrogenization in their ovaries compared to other women. Over 50 % of ovaries from women who were not BRCA1 mutation carriers had signs of estrogenization. The authors proposed that premature menopause is associated with loss of estrogen, which may lead to increased gonadotropin release via negative feedback. This in turn may promote carcinogenesis. Earlier menopause in BRCA1 mutation carriers was also observed, with mean age in BRCA carriers of 45.5 compared with 48.2 in noncarriers ($p < 0.05$).

7.5.1 Chemotherapy-Induced Amenorrhea

Chemotherapy may cause transient and reversible or permanent damage to the oocyte pool and ovarian reserve. This depends on the chemotherapy agent and dose, the preexisting ovarian reserve, and the age of the woman [113]. Effects of cytotoxic treatment, DNA damage, and apoptotic pathways on antral and dormant primordial follicles, as well as dormant primordial follicles, have been described [114].

The risk of amenorrhea after chemotherapy has been proposed to be higher in women with BRCA mutation, due to increased sensitivity of the ovarian follicles and higher risk of depletion [94]. Chemotherapy causes DNA damage, which the cell tries to repair. Multiple unrepaired DSBs then lead to apoptosis in growing follicles. In women with BRCA1 mutations, the lack of DSB repair will be even greater, increasing the risk of amenorrhea after chemotherapy [98].

Valentini et al. examined the risk of long-term amenorrhoea after chemotherapy, defined as absent menses beginning within 2 years of starting treatment and continuing for at least 2 years [89]. They compared BRCA1 and BRCA2 mutation carriers with a small group of noncarriers, who underwent chemotherapy. The results presented showed that BRCA mutation carriers did not have increased risk of amenorrhea. Women who experienced resumption of menses underwent menopause 3.6 years earlier if they underwent chemotherapy compared with those not receiving chemotherapy (45.4 vs 49.0, $p < 0.001$). The probability of chemotherapy-induced amenorrhea was significantly higher for BRCA2 carriers than for BRCA1 carriers (46.8 % v 32.7 %; $p < 0.001$), with early age of onset of amenorrhea in BRCA2 carriers. However, the conclusions of this study are somewhat dubious. The control group was very small compared to the BRCA1 carriers, and these women were treated with tamoxifen, which may also cause amenorrhea. Women underwent chemotherapy treatment 62 centers, and the details of chemotherapy are not presented. Further research is required to validate these findings.

One final important consideration is that platinum agents are considered particularly gonadotoxic [4] and there is an increasing trend for use of platinum agents among BC patients harboring a BRCA1/2 mutation, which may augment gonadotoxicity during neo-adjuvant/adjuvant chemotherapy.

7.6   Diminished Ovarian Reserve in BRCA Mutation Carriers

The link between diminished ovarian reserve in BRCA mutation carriers has been investigated in several studies, ranging from observation of ovarian reserve tests [95, 115], response and outcomes in in vitro fertilization (IVF) treatments [94, 116], patient-reported fertility [91, 97], and natural fertility in the absence of contraception [117].

A multicenter study examined parity and fertility in BRCA mutation carriers and noncarrier relatives [91]. No differences were observed in age at first birth, age at last birth, parity, or infertility. In a study of women of Ashkenazi Jewish descent with ovarian cancer, and without ovarian cancer, the association between BRCA mutation status and self-reported fertility, pregnancy rate, and pregnancy success was compared [91]. The study also examined sex ratio in the children born to these women. No difference was observed regarding fertility.

Conception and fertility in the context of "natural fertility conditions" was explored in a case-control study of woman in Utah [118]. The original BRCA mutation carriers served as probands to trace additional presumed carriers in their ancestors, based on the family pedigree as recorded in comprehensive state health records.

Controls were identified as women who had no familial connection to the BRCA carriers and presumed to be BRCA negative. According to their analysis, putative BRCA mutation carriers born prior to 1930 had significantly larger families, shorter spaces between births, and later age at last birth. These findings are similar, but not statistically significant, in women born after 1930.

Several recently published studies of ovarian reserve in BRCA mutation carriers presented conflicting results. Wang et al. [95] compared BRCA1 carriers, BRCA2 carriers and controls who were not carriers of a mutation, for Anti-Mullerian Hormone (AMH), considered the best single test for ovarian reserve testing [119]. Results were adjusted for age and BMI. BRCA1 mutation carriers had significantly lower AMH levels compared with controls (0.53 ng/mL [95 % confidence interval (CI) 0.33–0.77 ng/mL] vs. 1.05 ng/mL [95 % CI 0.76–1.40 ng/mL]). Logistic regression validated this finding: BRCA1 carriers had a fourfold increased odds of having AMH <1 ng/mL compared with controls (odds ratio 4.22, 95 % CI 1.48–12.0). No difference was observed in AMH levels between BRCA2 carriers and controls.

Conversely, Michaelson-Cohen et al. [115] tested BRCA1 and BRCA2 mutation carriers for AMH and found no significant difference in results compared with general population controls. This study did not examine BRCA1 and BRCA2 mutation carriers as distinct groups, and controls were from the general population, with no family history of BC.

Oktay et al. [94] reported their results of women with BC undergoing the COSTLESS protocol (Letrozole and Gonadotropin) for fertility preservation [120]. BRCA mutation testing was performed parallel to the treatment cycle, but results were only available after treatment was completed. Low ovarian response was defined as four or less oocytes retrieved in women younger than 38 years. Low ovarian response was significantly higher in women with BRCA mutation compared with no mutation (33.3 % vs 3.3 %; $p=0.014$) and BRCA-untested women (2.9 % $p=0.012$). Mean oocyte numbers were also significantly lower in women with BRCA mutation compared with BRCA mutation–negative women. BRCA1, but not BRCA2, mutations were associated with low response with an OR of 38.3 (95 % CI, 4.1–353.4; $p<0.001$).

A recent multicenter study [116] analyzed two groups of women with BRCA undergoing IVF. BRCA mutation–positive BC patients undergoing fertility preservation were compared with BRCA mutation negative or unknown breast cancer patients. BRCA mutation carriers undergoing IVF-PGD were compared with women undergoing IVF for male factor infertility, as well as women undergoing IVF-PGD for other reasons (not affecting ovarian reserve). Low response was defined as four or less oocytes retrieved. There was no significant difference in low response rate (8.77 % vs 8.46 %, $p=1$), number of oocytes retrieved (15.00 ± 8.06 vs. 14 ± 8.24, $p=0.44$), or number of 2PN embryos (9.61 ± 5.91 vs. 8.17 ± 5.55, $p=0.077$). Subgroup analysis according to age was also performed, with no observed differences. This study refutes the concept of diminished ovarian reserve, poorer response to treatment in BRCA mutation carriers, and BRCA positive women with BC.

7.7 Fertility Preservation and Preimplantation Genetic Diagnosis (PGD) for BRCA Mutation Carriers

7.7.1 Fertility Preservation Protocols for Women with BRCA Mutations

At the time of BC diagnosis many women have not yet completed their family, and some have not even commenced. During chemotherapy treatment, and resultant effect on ovarian reserve, and recommended 2-year postponement of conception following treatment [121], the remaining window of opportunity for childbearing may be limited. In women who are carriers of BRCA1/2 mutation, the recommendation for RRSO at completion of childbearing adds further time constraints [88]. Women diagnosed with BC are increasingly referred for consultation with fertility specialists prior to commencing potentially gonadotoxic chemotherapy [122, 123].

All young women with BC, irrespective of BRCA mutation status, should be offered thorough counseling regarding options for fertility preservation.

Fertility preservation options include embryo cryopreservation, oocyte cryopreservation, and oocyte tissue cryopreservation [124]. Ovarian stimulation protocols based on letrozole alone or in combination with gonadotropin result in lower serum estradiol levels than conventional IVF protocols and are favored by some [120]; however, tamoxifen-based protocols have been demonstrated to be safe and highly effective in a recent study by Meirow et al. [125].

There appears to be no additional risk of developing BC in women with BRCA mutations, who have experienced infertility, or undergone fertility treatment [96].

7.8 Preimplantation Genetic Diagnosis (PGD) and Prenatal Diagnosis for BRCA Mutation Carriers

Carriers of BRCA1/2 mutations have a 50 % chance of transmitting the mutation with each pregnancy, assuming their partner is BRCA mutation negative. Women who prefer to have children who will not be carriers of BRCA mutations may choose diagnosis during preimplantation and prenatal stages.

Prenatal diagnosis involves invasive tests which sample either the chorionic villi (CVS) or amniotic fluid (amniocentesis) in order to test karyotype abnormalities, or the presence or absence of single gene disorders. BRCA mutations may be tested by CVS or amniocentesis. A newer alternative is noninvasive prenatal testing, which tests cell-free DNA in maternal blood; however, this method is not yet available for BRCA mutation detection. Prenatal testing assists parents who may be considering termination of pregnancy for an affected fetus.

PGD is a technique offered to test embryos, usually on the third day following in vitro fertilization (IVF) [126]. Testing is performed on 1–2 cells of the developing embryo, usually at the blastomere stage. This allows for the selection of a healthy embryo for transfer. PGD was initially used for lethal or very severe genetic illnesses, but its use has been expanded to include disease carrier states. PGD is offered in many centers worldwide for BRCA1/2 mutations [127–129].

The timing of discussing the option of PGD is complex, as some women need time to comprehend and deal with the impact of BRCA mutation diagnosis, without being overwhelmed with more choices [130]. PGD is often raised as part of initial counseling for genetic testing for BRCA mutation. Recommendations of the National Society of Genetic Counselors' regarding broaching the option of PGD for women with BRCA1/2 mutation during genetic counseling, include providing as "much information as possible while acting in an ethical context that minimizes harm to clients and their families" [131].

Many women with BRCA mutations express concern about their current or future children [132] and are supportive of PGD as an option; however, the majority of women would not necessarily choose to take advantage of the existing technology for future pregnancies [132, 133]. PGD may provide an acceptable option for women who may have otherwise preferred not to risk having a natural biological child [134]. However, choosing PGD raises several challenging ethical issues, including the implications on the value of the life of the women carrying the mutation, as she herself may not have been born had the technology been available [135, 136]. PGD is also expensive and requires invasive, and possibly risky, medical treatment traditionally used in couples with infertility, when no actual fertility problem may exist.

The option of PGD should be presented with sensitivity given the complicated psychological and ethical issues, but is an important part of counseling and treatment of the BRCA mutation carrier.

7.9 Ovarian Tissue Cryopreservation for Fertility Preservation in Women with BRCA Mutation

More than 30 babies have been born following autotransplantation of cryopreserved ovarian tissue for fertility preservation [137, 138]. Ovarian tissue cryopreservation (OTC) is a form of fertility preservation which may be offered in conjunction with embryo or oocyte cryopreservation, or alone in prepubertal girls and young women. In women who need to start chemotherapy immediately, with no available window of opportunity for ovarian stimulation and oocyte harvesting or IVF, OTC may be offered without delaying cancer treatment. It can be performed at any stage of the menstrual cycle, does not involve exposure to hormones, and may be preferable in certain malignancies [138].

Autotransplantation of ovarian tissue carries potential risks of reintroducing malignancy, as ovarian grafts may harbor cancer cells [139]. In women with leukemia, disease recurrence following transplantation of cryopreserved ovarian tissue has been reported [140, 141].

Several studies found no evidence of malignant cell contamination of ovarian tissue in women with breast cancer [142, 143]. A review of literature regarding the safety of OTC in women with malignancy considered BC patients to be at low risk of recurrence following autotransplantation [144]. Bastings et al. [145] reviewed studies of ovarian metastases in ovarian tissue sampled. No metastases were identified in women with BC. Cancer recurrence was cited in one case of a BC survivor, although it is unclear if the recurrence was related to the transplantation [142].

No studies address BRCA mutation carriers specifically; however, the high risk of ovarian cancer in these women means that the risk of malignancy with reintroducing ovarian tissue would be higher than BC patients not carrying a mutation. While the risk of ovarian cancer in women with BRCA mutation is lower in women younger than 40, there have been no reports of women with BRCA mutation who underwent OTC. Thus the efficacy and safety of this method of fertility preservation remains unclear and is not an accepted practice in most centers for women harboring a BRCA mutation.

Conclusion

The presence of a BRCA1/2 mutation compounds the already complex and multifactorial challenges that exist when managing a young woman with breast cancer – the challenges range from medical (oncological, gynecological, surgical) to psychosocial and ethical; thus, a multidisciplinary approach is mandatory.

References

1. Collaborative Group on Hormonal Factors in Breast Cancer. Familial breast cancer: collaborative reanalysis of individual data from 52 epidemiological studies including 58,209 women with breast cancer and 101,986 women without the disease. Lancet. 2001;358(9291):1389–99.
2. Fletcher O, Houlston RS. Architecture of inherited susceptibility to common cancer. Nat Rev Cancer. 2010;10(5):353–61.
3. Cox A, et al. A common coding variant in CASP8 is associated with breast cancer risk. Nat Genet. 2007;39(3):352–8.
4. Meirow D, Nugent D. The effects of radiotherapy and chemotherapy on female reproduction. Hum Reprod Update. 2001;7(6):535–43.
5. Levy-Lahad E, et al. Founder BRCA1 and BRCA2 mutations in Ashkenazi Jews in Israel: frequency and differential penetrance in ovarian cancer and in breast-ovarian cancer families. Am J Hum Genet. 1997;60(5):1059–67.
6. Antoniou A, et al. Average risks of breast and ovarian cancer associated with BRCA1 or BRCA2 mutations detected in case Series unselected for family history: a combined analysis of 22 studies. Am J Hum Genet. 2003;72(5):1117–30.
7. Ford D, et al. Risks of cancer in BRCA1-mutation carriers. Breast Cancer Linkage Consortium Lancet. 1994;343(8899):692–5.
8. King MC, et al. Breast and ovarian cancer risks due to inherited mutations in BRCA1 and BRCA2. Science. 2003;302(5645):643–6.
9. Mavaddat N, et al. Cancer risks for BRCA1 and BRCA2 mutation carriers: results from prospective analysis of EMBRACE. J Natl Cancer Inst. 2013;105(11):812–22.
10. Zhang J, Powell SN. The role of the BRCA1 tumor suppressor in DNA double-strand break repair. Mol Cancer Res. 2005;3(10):531–9.
11. Moynahan ME, Pierce AJ, Jasin M. BRCA2 is required for homology-directed repair of chromosomal breaks. Mol Cell. 2001;7(2):263–72.
12. Golshan M, et al. The prevalence of germline BRCA1 and BRCA2 mutations in young women with breast cancer undergoing breast-conservation therapy. Am J Surg. 2006;192(1):58–62.

13. Peto J, et al. Prevalence of BRCA1 and BRCA2 gene mutations in patients with early-onset breast cancer. J Natl Cancer Inst. 1999;91(11):943–9.
14. Neuhausen S, et al. Recurrent BRCA2 6174delT mutations in Ashkenazi Jewish women affected by breast cancer. Nat Genet. 1996;13(1):126–8.
15. Offit K, et al. Germline BRCA1 185delAG mutations in Jewish women with breast cancer. Lancet. 1996;347(9016):1643–5.
16. Struewing JP, et al. The risk of cancer associated with specific mutations of BRCA1 and BRCA2 among Ashkenazi Jews. N Engl J Med. 1997;336(20):1401–8.
17. Rebbeck TR, Kauff ND, Domchek SM. Meta-analysis of risk reduction estimates associated with risk-reducing salpingo-oophorectomy in BRCA1 or BRCA2 mutation carriers. J Natl Cancer Inst. 2009;101(2):80–7.
18. Kauff ND, et al. Risk-reducing salpingo-oophorectomy in women with a BRCA1 or BRCA2 mutation. N Engl J Med. 2002;346(21):1609–15.
19. Rebbeck TR, et al. Prophylactic oophorectomy in carriers of BRCA1 or BRCA2 mutations. N Engl J Med. 2002;346(21):1616–22.
20. Rebbeck TR, et al. Breast cancer risk after bilateral prophylactic oophorectomy in BRCA1 mutation carriers. J Natl Cancer Inst. 1999;91(17):1475–9.
21. Eisen A, et al. Breast cancer risk following bilateral oophorectomy in BRCA1 and BRCA2 mutation carriers: an international case-control study. J Clin Oncol. 2005;23(30):7491–6.
22. Genetic/familial high risk assessment: breast & ovarian. National Comprehensive Cancer Network.
23. Robson M, et al. Breast conservation therapy for invasive breast cancer in Ashkenazi women with BRCA gene founder mutations. J Natl Cancer Inst. 1999;91(24):2112–7.
24. Warner E, et al. Surveillance of BRCA1 and BRCA2 mutation carriers with magnetic resonance imaging, ultrasound, mammography, and clinical breast examination. JAMA. 2004; 292(11):1317–25.
25. Veronesi A, et al. Familial breast cancer: characteristics and outcome of BRCA 1-2 positive and negative cases. BMC Cancer. 2005;5:70.
26. Lakhani SR, et al. The pathology of familial breast cancer: predictive value of immunohistochemical markers estrogen receptor, progesterone receptor, HER-2, and p53 in patients with mutations in BRCA1 and BRCA2. J Clin Oncol. 2002;20(9):2310–8.
27. Atchley DP, et al. Clinical and pathologic characteristics of patients with BRCA-positive and BRCA-negative breast cancer. J Clin Oncol. 2008;26(26):4282–8.
28. Rennert G, et al. Clinical outcomes of breast cancer in carriers of BRCA1 and BRCA2 mutations. N Engl J Med. 2007;357(2):115–23.
29. Huzarski T, et al. Ten-year survival in patients with BRCA1-negative and BRCA1-positive breast cancer. J Clin Oncol. 2013;31(26):3191–6.
30. Robson ME, et al. A combined analysis of outcome following breast cancer: differences in survival based on BRCA1/BRCA2 mutation status and administration of adjuvant treatment. Breast Cancer Res. 2004;6(1):R8–17.
31. Goodwin PJ, et al. Breast cancer prognosis in BRCA1 and BRCA2 mutation carriers: an International Prospective Breast Cancer Family Registry population-based cohort study. J Clin Oncol. 2012;30(1):19–26.
32. Bayraktar S, et al. Outcome of triple-negative breast cancer in patients with or without deleterious BRCA mutations. Breast Cancer Res Treat. 2011;130(1):145–53.
33. Lee E, et al. Characteristics of triple-negative breast cancer in patients with a BRCA1 mutation: results from a population-based study of young women. J Clin Oncol. 2011;29(33): 4373–80.
34. Abbott DW, Freeman ML, Holt JT. Double-strand break repair deficiency and radiation sensitivity in BRCA2 mutant cancer cells. J Natl Cancer Inst. 1998;90(13):978–85.
35. Farmer H, et al. Targeting the DNA repair defect in BRCA mutant cells as a therapeutic strategy. Nature. 2005;434(7035):917–21.
36. Tutt AN, et al. Exploiting the DNA repair defect in BRCA mutant cells in the design of new therapeutic strategies for cancer. Cold Spring Harb Symp Quant Biol. 2005;70:139–48.

37. Tassone P, et al. BRCA1 expression modulates chemosensitivity of BRCA1-defective HCC1937 human breast cancer cells. Br J Cancer. 2003;88(8):1285–91.
38. Quinn JE, et al. BRCA1 functions as a differential modulator of chemotherapy-induced apoptosis. Cancer Res. 2003;63(19):6221–8.
39. Kennedy RD, et al. The role of BRCA1 in the cellular response to chemotherapy. J Natl Cancer Inst. 2004;96(22):1659–68.
40. Foulkes WD. BRCA1 and BRCA2: chemosensitivity, treatment outcomes and prognosis. Fam Cancer. 2006;5(2):135–42.
41. Kriege M, et al. Sensitivity to first-line chemotherapy for metastatic breast cancer in BRCA1 and BRCA2 mutation carriers. J Clin Oncol. 2009;27(23):3764–71.
42. Chalasani P, Livingston R. Differential chemotherapeutic sensitivity for breast tumors with "BRCAness": a review. Oncologist. 2013;18(8):909–16.
43. Bayraktar S, Gluck S. Systemic therapy options in BRCA mutation-associated breast cancer. Breast Cancer Res Treat. 2013;135(2):355–66.
44. Byrski T, et al. Pathologic complete response rates in young women with BRCA1-positive breast cancers after neoadjuvant chemotherapy. J Clin Oncol. 2010;28(3):375–9.
45. Byrski T, et al. Results of a phase II open-label, non-randomized trial of cisplatin chemotherapy in patients with BRCA1-positive metastatic breast cancer. Breast Cancer Res. 2014;14(4):R110.
46. Silver DP, et al. Efficacy of neoadjuvant Cisplatin in triple-negative breast cancer. J Clin Oncol. 2010;28(7):1145–53.
47. Wysocki PJ, et al. Primary resistance to docetaxel-based chemotherapy in metastatic breast cancer patients correlates with a high frequency of BRCA1 mutations. Med Sci Monit. 2008;14(7):SC7–10.
48. Byrski T, et al. Response to neo-adjuvant chemotherapy in women with BRCA1-positive breast cancers. Breast Cancer Res Treat. 2008;108(2):289–96.
49. Kriege M, et al. The efficacy of taxane chemotherapy for metastatic breast cancer in BRCA1 and BRCA2 mutation carriers. Cancer. 2012;118(4):899–907.
50. Anders CK, et al. Poly(ADP-Ribose) polymerase inhibition: "targeted" therapy for triple-negative breast cancer. Clin Cancer Res. 2010;16(19):4702–10.
51. Fong PC, et al. Inhibition of poly(ADP-ribose) polymerase in tumors from BRCA mutation carriers. N Engl J Med. 2009;361(2):123–34.
52. Tutt A, et al. Oral poly(ADP-ribose) polymerase inhibitor olaparib in patients with BRCA1 or BRCA2 mutations and advanced breast cancer: a proof-of-concept trial. Lancet. 2010;376(9737):235–44.
53. Friebel TM, Domchek SM, Rebbeck TR. Modifiers of cancer risk in BRCA1 and BRCA2 mutation carriers: systematic review and meta-analysis. J Natl Cancer Inst. 2014;106(6):dju091.
54. Chin J, Konje JC, Hickey M. Levonorgestrel intrauterine system for endometrial protection in women with breast cancer on adjuvant tamoxifen. Cochrane Database Syst Rev. 2009;(4):CD007245.
55. Shi Q, et al. The role of levonorgestrel-releasing intrauterine system for endometrial protection in women with breast cancer taking tamoxifen. Eur J Gynaecol Oncol. 2014;35(5):492–8.
56. Fu Y, Zhuang Z. Long-term effects of levonorgestrel-releasing intrauterine system on tamoxifen-treated breast cancer patients: a meta-analysis. Int J Clin Exp Pathol. 2014;7(10):6419–29.
57. Trinh XB, et al. Use of the levonorgestrel-releasing intrauterine system in breast cancer patients. Fertil Steril. 2008;90(1):17–22.
58. Lyytinen HK, et al. A case-control study on hormone therapy as a risk factor for breast cancer in Finland: Intrauterine system carries a risk as well. Int J Cancer. 2010;126(2):483–9.
59. Kwon JS, et al. Prophylactic salpingectomy and delayed oophorectomy as an alternative for BRCA mutation carriers. Obstet Gynecol. 2013;121(1):14–24.
60. Schenberg T, Mitchell G. Prophylactic bilateral salpingectomy as a prevention strategy in women at high-risk of ovarian cancer: a mini-review. Front Oncol. 2014;4:21.

61. Charlton BM, et al. Oral contraceptive use and mortality after 36 years of follow-up in the Nurses' Health Study: prospective cohort study. BMJ. 2014;349:g6356.
62. Bernholtz S, et al. Cancer risk in Jewish BRCA1 and BRCA2 mutation carriers: effects of oral contraceptive use and parental origin of mutation. Breast Cancer Res Treat. 2011; 129(2):557–63.
63. Cibula D, et al. Oral contraceptives and risk of ovarian and breast cancers in BRCA mutation carriers: a meta-analysis. Expert Rev Anticancer Ther. 2011;11(8):1197–207.
64. Jernstrom H, et al. Impact of teenage oral contraceptive use in a population-based series of early-onset breast cancer cases who have undergone BRCA mutation testing. Eur J Cancer. 2005;41(15):2312–20.
65. Kotsopoulos J, et al. Timing of oral contraceptive use and the risk of breast cancer in BRCA1 mutation carriers. Breast Cancer Res Treat. 2014;143(3):579–86.
66. Gadducci A, et al. Gynaecologic challenging issues in the management of BRCA mutation carriers: oral contraceptives, prophylactic salpingo-oophorectomy and hormone replacement therapy. Gynecol Endocrinol. 2010;26(8):568–77.
67. Narod SA, et al. Oral contraceptives and the risk of breast cancer in BRCA1 and BRCA2 mutation carriers. J Natl Cancer Inst. 2002;94(23):1773–9.
68. Iodice S, et al. Oral contraceptive use and breast or ovarian cancer risk in BRCA1/2 carriers: a meta-analysis. Eur J Cancer. 2010;46(12):2275–84.
69. Moorman PG, et al. Oral contraceptives and risk of ovarian cancer and breast cancer among high-risk women: a systematic review and meta-analysis. J Clin Oncol. 2013;31(33): 4188–98.
70. Grenader T, et al. BRCA1 and BRCA2 germ-line mutations and oral contraceptives: to use or not to use. Breast. 2005;14(4):264–8.
71. Lee E, et al. Effect of reproductive factors and oral contraceptives on breast cancer risk in BRCA1/2 mutation carriers and noncarriers: results from a population-based study. Cancer Epidemiol Biomarkers Prev. 2008;17(11):3170–8.
72. Haile RW, et al. BRCA1 and BRCA2 mutation carriers, oral contraceptive use, and breast cancer before age 50. Cancer Epidemiol Biomarkers Prev. 2006;15(10):1863–70.
73. Milne RL, et al. Oral contraceptive use and risk of early-onset breast cancer in carriers and noncarriers of BRCA1 and BRCA2 mutations. Cancer Epidemiol Biomarkers Prev. 2005;14(2):350–6.
74. Althuis MD, et al. Breast cancers among very young premenopausal women (United States). Cancer Causes Control. 2003;14(2):151–60.
75. Tavani A, et al. Risk factors for breast cancer in women under 40 years. Eur J Cancer. 1999;35(9):1361–7.
76. Kotsopoulos J, et al. Age at menarche and the risk of breast cancer in BRCA1 and BRCA2 mutation carriers. Cancer Causes Control. 2005;16(6):667–74.
77. Collaborative Group on Hormonal Factors in Breast Cancer. Breast cancer and breastfeeding: collaborative reanalysis of individual data from 47 epidemiological studies in 30 countries, including 50302 women with breast cancer and 96973 women without the disease. Lancet. 2002;360(9328):187–95.
78. Clavel-Chapelon F, Gerber M. Reproductive factors and breast cancer risk. Do they differ according to age at diagnosis? Breast Cancer Res Treat. 2002;72(2):107–15.
79. Narod SA. Modifiers of risk of hereditary breast and ovarian cancer. Nat Rev Cancer. 2002;2(2):113–23.
80. Cullinane CA, et al. Effect of pregnancy as a risk factor for breast cancer in BRCA1/BRCA2 mutation carriers. Int J Cancer. 2005;117(6):988–91.
81. Andrieu N, et al. Pregnancies, breast-feeding, and breast cancer risk in the International BRCA1/2 Carrier Cohort Study (IBCCS). J Natl Cancer Inst. 2006;98(8):535–44.
82. Antoniou AC, et al. Parity and breast cancer risk among BRCA1 and BRCA2 mutation carriers. Breast Cancer Res. 2006;8(6):R72.
83. Milne RL, et al. Parity and the risk of breast and ovarian cancer in BRCA1 and BRCA2 mutation carriers. Breast Cancer Res Treat. 2010;119(1):221–32.

84. Pan H, et al. Reproductive factors and breast cancer risk among BRCA1 or BRCA2 mutation carriers: results from ten studies. Cancer Epidemiol. 2014;38(1):1–8.
85. Lecarpentier J, et al. Variation in breast cancer risk associated with factors related to pregnancies according to truncating mutation location, in the French National BRCA1 and BRCA2 mutations carrier cohort (GENEPSO). Breast Cancer Res. 2012;14(4):R99.
86. Jernstrom H, et al. Breast-feeding and the risk of breast cancer in BRCA1 and BRCA2 mutation carriers. J Natl Cancer Inst. 2004;96(14):1094–8.
87. Kotsopoulos J, et al. Breastfeeding and the risk of breast cancer in BRCA1 and BRCA2 mutation carriers. Breast Cancer Res. 2012;14(2):R42.
88. Finch A, Evans G, Narod SA. BRCA carriers, prophylactic salpingo-oophorectomy and menopause: clinical management considerations and recommendations. Womens Health (Lond Engl). 2012;8(5):543–55.
89. Valentini A, et al. Chemotherapy-induced amenorrhea in patients with breast cancer with a BRCA1 or BRCA2 mutation. J Clin Oncol. 2013;31(31):3914–9.
90. Tea MK, et al. Association of BRCA1/2 mutations with FMR1 genotypes: effects on menarcheal and menopausal age. Maturitas. 2013;75(2):148–51.
91. Pal T, et al. Fertility in women with BRCA mutations: a case-control study. Fertil Steril. 2010;93(6):1805–8.
92. Finch A, et al. Frequency of premature menopause in women who carry a BRCA1 or BRCA2 mutation. Fertil Steril. 2013;99(6):1724–8.
93. Lin WT, et al. Comparison of age at natural menopause in BRCA1/2 mutation carriers with a non-clinic-based sample of women in northern California. Cancer. 2013;119(9):1652–9.
94. Oktay K, et al. Association of BRCA1 mutations with occult primary ovarian insufficiency: a possible explanation for the link between infertility and breast/ovarian cancer risks. J Clin Oncol. 2010;28(2):240–4.
95. Wang ET, et al. BRCA1 germline mutations may be associated with reduced ovarian reserve. Fertil Steril. 2014;102(6):1723–8.
96. Kotsopoulos J, et al. Infertility, treatment of infertility, and the risk of breast cancer among women with BRCA1 and BRCA2 mutations: a case-control study. Cancer Causes Control. 2008;19(10):1111–9.
97. Moslehi R, et al. Impact of BRCA mutations on female fertility and offspring sex ratio. Am J Hum Biol. 2010;22(2):201–5.
98. Oktay K, et al. Age-related decline in DNA repair function explains diminished ovarian reserve, earlier menopause, and possible oocyte vulnerability to chemotherapy in women with BRCA mutations. J Clin Oncol. 2014;32(10):1093–4.
99. French JD, et al. Disruption of BRCA1 function results in telomere lengthening and increased anaphase bridge formation in immortalized cell lines. Genes Chromosomes Cancer. 2006;45(3):277–89.
100. McPherson JP, et al. A role for Brca1 in chromosome end maintenance. Hum Mol Genet. 2006;15(6):831–8.
101. Bau DT, et al. Breast cancer risk and the DNA double-strand break end-joining capacity of nonhomologous end-joining genes are affected by BRCA1. Cancer Res. 2004;64(14):5013–9.
102. Zhong Q, et al. BRCA1 facilitates microhomology-mediated end joining of DNA double strand breaks. J Biol Chem. 2002;277(32):28641–7.
103. Bae I, et al. BRCA1 induces antioxidant gene expression and resistance to oxidative stress. Cancer Res. 2004;64(21):7893–909.
104. Titus S, et al. Impairment of BRCA1-related DNA double-strand break repair leads to ovarian aging in mice and humans. Sci Transl Med. 2013;5(172):172ra21.
105. Giscard d'Estaing S, et al. Upregulation of the BRCA1 gene in human germ cells and in preimplantation embryos. Fertil Steril. 2005;84(3):785–8.
106. Gleicher N, Weghofer A, Barad DH. Ovarian reserve determinations suggest new function of FMR1 (fragile X gene) in regulating ovarian ageing. Reprod Biomed Online. 2010;20(6):768–75.

107. Brandao RD, et al. FMR1 low sub-genotype does not rescue BRCA1/2-mutated human embryos and does not explain primary ovarian insufficiency among BRCA1/2-carriers. Hum Reprod. 2013;28(8):2308–11.
108. Prostaglandins and abortion. I. intramuscular administration of 15-methyl prostaglandin F2alpha for induction of abortion in weeks 10 to 20 of pregnancy. World Health Organization Task Force on the Use of Prostaglandins for the Regulation of Fertility. Am J Obstet Gynecol. 1977;129(6):593–6.
109. Fortuno C, Labarta E. Genetics of primary ovarian insufficiency: a review. J Assist Reprod Genet. 2014;31(12):1573–85.
110. Cox L, Liu JH. Primary ovarian insufficiency: an update. Int J Womens Health. 2014;6: 235–43.
111. Collins IM, et al. Do BRCA1 and BRCA2 mutation carriers have earlier natural menopause than their noncarrier relatives? Results from the Kathleen Cuningham Foundation Consortium for Research into Familial Breast Cancer. J Clin Oncol. 2013;31(31):3920–5.
112. Rzepka-Gorska I, et al. Premature menopause in patients with BRCA1 gene mutation. Breast Cancer Res Treat. 2006;100(1):59–63.
113. Fusek M, Lin XL, Tang J. Enzymic properties of thermopsin. J Biol Chem. 1990;265(3): 1496–501.
114. Roness H, Kalich-Philosoph L, Meirow D. Prevention of chemotherapy-induced ovarian damage: possible roles for hormonal and non-hormonal attenuating agents. Hum Reprod Update. 2014;20(5):759–74.
115. Michaelson-Cohen R, et al. BRCA mutation carriers do not have compromised ovarian reserve. Int J Gynecol Cancer. 2014;24(2):233–7.
116. Meirow D, Eldar-Geva T, Manela D, Brenghausen M, Shapira M, Raanani H. BRCA mutation carriers do not show reduced ovarian reserve as demonstrated by IVF treatments outcome, in ASRM. Fertil Steril: Honolulu; 2014.
117. Smith KR, et al. Effects of BRCA1 and BRCA2 mutations on female fertility. Proc Biol Sci. 2012;279(1732):1389–95.
118. Smith KR, Hanson HA, Hollingshaus MS. BRCA1 and BRCA2 mutations and female fertility. Curr Opin Obstet Gynecol. 2013;25(3):207–13.
119. Broer SL, et al. Anti-Mullerian hormone: ovarian reserve testing and its potential clinical implications. Hum Reprod Update. 2014;20(5):688–701.
120. Rodriguez-Wallberg KA, Oktay K. Fertility preservation in women with breast cancer. Clin Obstet Gynecol. 2010;53(4):753–62.
121. Meirow D, et al. Toxicity of chemotherapy and radiation on female reproduction. Clin Obstet Gynecol. 2010;53(4):727–39.
122. Adams E, Hill E, Watson E. Fertility preservation in cancer survivors: a national survey of oncologists' current knowledge, practice and attitudes. Br J Cancer. 2013;108(8):1602–15.
123. Munster PN. Fertility preservation and breast cancer: a complex problem. Oncology (Williston Park). 2013;27(6):533–9.
124. Moffat R, Guth U. Preserving fertility in patients undergoing treatment for breast cancer: current perspectives. Breast Cancer (Dove Med Press). 2014;6:93–101.
125. Meirow D, et al. Tamoxifen co-administration during controlled ovarian hyperstimulation for in vitro fertilization in breast cancer patients increases the safety of fertility-preservation treatment strategies. Fertil Steril. 2014;102(2):488–95 e3.
126. Basille C, et al. Preimplantation genetic diagnosis: state of the art. Eur J Obstet Gynecol Reprod Biol. 2009;145(1):9–13.
127. Sagi M, et al. Preimplantation genetic diagnosis for BRCA1/2–a novel clinical experience. Prenat Diagn. 2009;29(5):508–13.
128. Derks-Smeets IA, et al. Hereditary breast and ovarian cancer and reproduction: an observational study on the suitability of preimplantation genetic diagnosis for both asymptomatic carriers and breast cancer survivors. Breast Cancer Res Treat. 2014;145(3):673–81.
129. Ramon YCT, et al. Preimplantation genetic diagnosis for inherited breast cancer: first clinical application and live birth in Spain. Fam Cancer. 2012;11(2):175–9.

130. Hurley K, et al. Incorporating information regarding preimplantation genetic diagnosis into discussions concerning testing and risk management for BRCA1/2 mutations: a qualitative study of patient preferences. Cancer. 2012;118(24):6270–7.
131. Berliner JL, Fay AM, Practice Issues Subcommittee of the National Society of Genetic Counselors' Familial Cancer Risk Counseling Special Interest Group. Risk assessment and genetic counseling for hereditary breast and ovarian cancer: recommendations of the National Society of Genetic Counselors. J Genet Couns. 2007;16(3):241–60.
132. Staton AD, et al. Cancer risk reduction and reproductive concerns in female BRCA1/2 mutation carriers. Fam Cancer. 2008;7(2):179–86.
133. Menon U, et al. Views of BRCA gene mutation carriers on preimplantation genetic diagnosis as a reproductive option for hereditary breast and ovarian cancer. Hum Reprod. 2007;22(6):1573–7.
134. Smith KR, et al. Fertility intentions following testing for a BRCA1 gene mutation. Cancer Epidemiol Biomarkers Prev. 2004;13(5):733–40.
135. Quinn GP, et al. Conflict between values and technology: perceptions of preimplantation genetic diagnosis among women at increased risk for hereditary breast and ovarian cancer. Fam Cancer. 2009;8(4):441–9.
136. Ormondroyd E, et al. Attitudes to reproductive genetic testing in women who had a positive BRCA test before having children: a qualitative analysis. Eur J Hum Genet. 2012;20(1):4–10.
137. Meirow D, Ra'anani H, Biderman H. Ovarian tissue cryopreservation and transplantation: a realistic, effective technology for fertility preservation. Methods Mol Biol. 2014;1154:455–73.
138. Gamzatova Z, et al. Autotransplantation of cryopreserved ovarian tissue–effective method of fertility preservation in cancer patients. Gynecol Endocrinol. 2014;30 Suppl 1:43–7.
139. Meirow D, et al. Searching for evidence of disease and malignant cell contamination in ovarian tissue stored from hematologic cancer patients. Hum Reprod. 2008;23(5):1007–13.
140. Dolmans MM, et al. Reimplantation of cryopreserved ovarian tissue from patients with acute lymphoblastic leukemia is potentially unsafe. Blood. 2010;116(16):2908–14.
141. Rosendahl M, et al. Evidence of residual disease in cryopreserved ovarian cortex from female patients with leukemia. Fertil Steril. 2010;94(6):2186–90.
142. Rosendahl M, et al. Cryopreservation of ovarian tissue for fertility preservation: no evidence of malignant cell contamination in ovarian tissue from patients with breast cancer. Fertil Steril. 2011;95(6):2158–61.
143. Sanchez-Serrano M, et al. Malignant cells are not found in ovarian cortex from breast cancer patients undergoing ovarian cortex cryopreservation. Hum Reprod. 2009;24(9):2238–43.
144. Rosendahl M, Greve T, Andersen CY. The safety of transplanting cryopreserved ovarian tissue in cancer patients: a review of the literature. J Assist Reprod Genet. 2013;30(1):11–24.
145. Bastings L, et al. Autotransplantation of cryopreserved ovarian tissue in cancer survivors and the risk of reintroducing malignancy: a systematic review. Hum Reprod Update. 2013;19(5):483–506.

Printed by Printforce, the Netherlands